RISK AND RESPONSIBILITY: THE ROLES OF FDA AND PHARMACEUTICAL COMPANIES IN ENSURING THE SAFETY OF APPROVED DRUGS, LIKE VIOXX

HEARING

BEFORE THE

COMMITTEE ON GOVERNMENT REFORM

HOUSE OF REPRESENTATIVES

ONE HUNDRED NINTH CONGRESS

FIRST SESSION

MAY 5, 2005

Serial No. 109–27

Printed for the use of the Committee on Government Reform

Available via the World Wide Web: http://www.gpo.gov/congress/house
http://www.house.gov/reform

U.S. GOVERNMENT PRINTING OFFICE

21–483 PDF   WASHINGTON : 2005

COMMITTEE ON GOVERNMENT REFORM

TOM DAVIS, Virginia, *Chairman*

CHRISTOPHER SHAYS, Connecticut
DAN BURTON, Indiana
ILEANA ROS-LEHTINEN, Florida
JOHN M. McHUGH, New York
JOHN L. MICA, Florida
GIL GUTKNECHT, Minnesota
MARK E. SOUDER, Indiana
STEVEN C. LaTOURETTE, Ohio
TODD RUSSELL PLATTS, Pennsylvania
CHRIS CANNON, Utah
JOHN J. DUNCAN, JR., Tennessee
CANDICE S. MILLER, Michigan
MICHAEL R. TURNER, Ohio
DARRELL E. ISSA, California
GINNY BROWN-WAITE, Florida
JON C. PORTER, Nevada
KENNY MARCHANT, Texas
LYNN A. WESTMORELAND, Georgia
PATRICK T. McHENRY, North Carolina
CHARLES W. DENT, Pennsylvania
VIRGINIA FOXX, North Carolina

HENRY A. WAXMAN, California
TOM LANTOS, California
MAJOR R. OWENS, New York
EDOLPHUS TOWNS, New York
PAUL E. KANJORSKI, Pennsylvania
CAROLYN B. MALONEY, New York
ELIJAH E. CUMMINGS, Maryland
DENNIS J. KUCINICH, Ohio
DANNY K. DAVIS, Illinois
WM. LACY CLAY, Missouri
DIANE E. WATSON, California
STEPHEN F. LYNCH, Massachusetts
CHRIS VAN HOLLEN, Maryland
LINDA T. SANCHEZ, California
C.A. DUTCH RUPPERSBERGER, Maryland
BRIAN HIGGINS, New York
ELEANOR HOLMES NORTON, District of
Columbia

———

BERNARD SANDERS, Vermont
(Independent)

MELISSA WOJCIAK, *Staff Director*
DAVID MARIN, *Deputy Staff Director/Communications Director*
ROB BORDEN, *Parliamentarian*
TERESA AUSTIN, *Chief Clerk*
PHIL BARNETT, *Minority Chief of Staff/Chief Counsel*

CONTENTS

RISK AND RESPONSIBILITY: THE ROLES OF FDA AND PHARMACEUTICAL COMPANIES IN ENSURING THE SAFETY OF APPROVED DRUGS, LIKE VIOXX

THURSDAY, MAY 5, 2005

House of Representatives,
Committee on Government Reform,
Washington, DC.

The Committee met, pursuant to notice, at 10:25 a.m., in room 2154, Rayburn House Office Building, Hon. Tom Davis of Virginia (chairman of the committee) presiding.

Present: Representatives Tom Davis, Mica, Gutknecht, Souder, Brown-Waite, Porter, Marchant, Westmoreland, Dent, Foxx, Waxman, Towns, Cummings, Kucinich, Watson, Van Hollen, Ruppersberger, and Higgins.

Staff present: David Marin, deputy staff director/communications director; Keith Ausbrook, chief counsel; Jennifer Safavian, chief counsel for oversight and investigations; Anne Marie Turner and Jim Moore, counsels; Rob White, press secretary; Drew Crockett, deputy director of communications; Susie Schulte and Mindi Walker, professional staff members; Randy Cole, GAO detailee; Teresa Austin, chief clerk; Sarah D'Orsie, deputy clerk; Allyson Blandford, office manager; Corinne Zaccagnini, chief information officer; Leneal Scott, computer systems manager; Todd Greenwood, staff assistant; Phil Barnett, minority staff director/chief counsel; Kristin Amerling, minority deputy chief counsel; Karen Lightfoot, minority communications director/senior policy advisor; Naomi Seller, minority counsel; Josh Sharfstein, minority professional staff member; Earley Green, minority chief clerk; Jean Gosa, minority assistant clerk; Christopher Davis, minority investigator; and Therese Foote, minority special assistant.

Chairman TOM DAVIS. The committee will come to order. I want to thank everybody for bearing with us through the markup.

The committee is here today to discuss the roles of the Food and Drug Administration and pharmaceutical companies in ensuring the safety of approved drugs. More specifically, we are going to examine the post-approval actions taken by the FDA and Merck and Co. related to the arthritis and acute pain medication Vioxx, and highlight concerns arising from our investigation into the relationship between offices within the FDA Center for Drug Evaluation and Research.

This committee's investigation began after Merck's September 30, 2004 voluntary world-wide withdrawal of Vioxx. The Vioxx re-

(1)

call came after 5 years on the market with Merck's annual sales for the drug topping $2.5 billion and more than 80 million patients having taken the drug. The decision to withdraw Vioxx was made after Merck's own clinical studies showed that 3½ percent of Vioxx takers suffered a heart attack or stroke, compared with 1.9 percent of patients taking a placebo. That study followed an earlier study that showed a significant disparity in heart attacks between those patients taking Vioxx and those taking naproxen, commonly sold as Aleve. The earlier study had resulted in the use of new labeling on Vioxx that had been in effect since April 2002.

After the Vioxx study and its ultimate withdrawal, other clinical trials raised serious questions about the cardiovascular risks associated with other Cox–2 inhibitors, such as Celebrex and Bextra and other non-steroidal anti-inflammatory drugs, such as naproxen. As a result, patients suffering from arthritis or acute pain were concerned and confused about choosing the proper pain medication.

In February 2004, the FDA convened an advisory committee meeting to address these concerns. On April 7, 2005, after reviewing the recommendations of the advisory committee, the FDA asked Pfizer to remove Bextra from the market, and to include a black box warning on Celebrex. The FDA made no official ruling or recommendation regarding Vioxx since Merck voluntarily removed it from the market.

This brings us to why we are here today. Most average Americans believe that once the FDA approves a drug, that drug carries the Good Housekeeping seal of approval. If this were the case, there would be no need for post-marketing surveillance of any drug. Due to the inability of any company to enlist millions of people to participate in preapproved trials, it is imperative that deliberate, post-approval surveillance take place and that doctors and pharmaceutical companies report to the FDA the adverse reactions to drugs.

As part of its investigation, the committee requested volumes of documents from and conducted hours of interviews with FDA and Merck regarding post-marketing surveillance. The information obtained has raised questions regarding Merck's knowledge of the cardiovascular risks of Vioxx based on its post-approval research and how Merck informed the public and physicians on the risk.

Merck employed over 3,000 field representatives for the marketing of Vioxx, did the training materials provided to Merck's sales force, adequately covered the cardiovascular risks for Vioxx? Based on those materials, were the representatives presenting a fair and balanced presentation to physicians on the safety of Vioxx? We are pleased to have Merck representatives here today, voluntarily, to answer these questions.

Our investigation also raised questions about the FDA's role in ensuring the safety of drugs after formal approval for sale to the public. Is there a need to strengthen FDA's role in updating safety warnings of previously approved drugs? How do we address these concerns without prematurely depriving millions of people of the benefits of the drug as already demonstrated?

As the committee conducted its investigation, it became apparent that the relationship between the Office of New Drugs and the Office of Drug Safety has its challenges. It appears that a lack of communication between the offices, as well as communication up the chain of command of these offices, has contributed to some discord within CDER.

We are pleased to have the Directors of CDER, of the Office of New Drugs and the Office of Drug Safety here to discuss the steps the FDA is taking to address interaction and coordination between the offices, including the creation of a drug safety monitoring board to monitor post-marketing risks and benefits of drugs.

We are not here today to point fingers. We are here to explore how drug companies and FDA can work together and independently to ensure the best possible post-marketing surveillance of drugs. We are here to ensure that FDA has taken the necessary actions to ensure better communications between the Office of New Drugs and the Office of Drugs Safety and that the public is informed regarding the safety of these drugs. Finally, we are here to examine Merck's responsibility in informing physicians and the public about the efficacy and safety of Vioxx.

I would now recognize the distinguished ranking member, Mr. Waxman, for his opening statement.

[The prepared statement of Chairman Tom Davis follows:]

Statement of Chairman Tom Davis
Risk and Responsibility: The Roles of FDA and Pharmaceutical
Companies in Ensuring the Safety of Approved Drugs, Like Vioxx
May 5, 2005

Good morning. The Committee is here today to discuss the roles of the Food and Drug Administration (FDA) and pharmaceutical companies in ensuring the safety of approved drugs. More specifically, we will examine the post-approval actions taken by FDA and Merck & Co., Inc. (Merck) related to the arthritis and acute pain medication, Vioxx, and highlight concerns arising from our investigation into the relationship between offices within FDA's Center for Drug Evaluation and Research.

This Committee's investigation began after Merck's September 30, 2004, voluntary world-wide withdrawal of Vioxx. The Vioxx recall came after 5 years on the market, with Merck's annual sales for the drug topping $2.5 billion, and more than 80 million patients having taken the drug. The decision to withdraw Vioxx was made after Merck's own clinical study showed that 3.5% of Vioxx takers suffered a heart attack or stroke, compared with 1.9% of patients taking a placebo. That study followed an earlier study that showed a significant disparity in heart attacks between those patients taking Vioxx and those taking naproxen (commonly sold as Aleve). The earlier study had resulted in the use of new labeling on Vioxx that had been in effect since April 2002.

After the Vioxx study and its ultimate withdrawal, other clinical trials raised serious questions about the cardiovascular risks associated with other COX-2 inhibitors, such as Celebrex and Bextra, and other nonsteroidal anti-inflammatory drugs, such as naproxen. As a result, patients suffering from arthritis or acute pain were concerned and confused about choosing the proper pain medication. In February 2004, the FDA convened an Advisory Committee meeting to address these concerns.

On April 7, 2005, after reviewing the recommendations of the Advisory Committee, FDA asked Pfizer to remove Bextra from the market and to include a "black box" warning on Celebrex. FDA made no official ruling or recommendation regarding Vioxx since Merck voluntarily removed it from the market.

This brings us to why we are here today. Most average Americans believe that once the FDA approves a drug, that drug carries the Good Housekeeping Seal of Approval. If this were the case, there would be no need for post-marketing surveillance of any drug. Due to the inability of any company to enlist millions of people to participate in pre-approval trials, it is imperative that deliberate post-approval surveillance takes place and that doctors and pharmaceutical companies report to the FDA the adverse reactions of drugs.

As part of its investigation, the Committee requested volumes of documents from and conducted hours of interviews with FDA and Merck regarding post-marketing surveillance. The information obtained has raised questions regarding Merck's knowledge of the cardiovascular risks of Vioxx based on its post-approval research, and how Merck informed the public and physicians of the risk. Merck employed over 3,000 field representatives for the marketing of Vioxx: – did the training materials provided to Merck's sales force adequately cover the cardiovascular risks for Vioxx? Based on those materials, were the representatives presenting a fair and balanced presentation to physicians on the safety of Vioxx? We are pleased to have a Merck representative here today, voluntarily, to answer these questions.

Our investigation also raised questions about the FDA's role in ensuring the safety of drugs after formal approval for sale to the public. Is there a need to strengthen FDA's role in updating safety warnings of previously approved drugs? How do we address these concerns without prematurely depriving millions of people of the benefits that the drug has already demonstrated.

As the Committee conducted its investigation, it became apparent that the relationship between the Office of New Drugs and the Office of Drug Safety has it challenges. It appears that a lack of communication between the offices, as well as communication up the chain of command of these offices has contributed to some discord within CDER (pronounced See-Der). We are pleased to have the Directors of CDER, Office of New Drugs, and Office of Drug Safety here to discuss the steps FDA is taking to address interaction and coordination between the offices, including the creation of the Drug Safety Monitoring Board to monitor post-marketing risks and benefits of drugs.

We aren't here today to point fingers. We are here to explore how drug companies and FDA can work together, and independently, to ensure the best possible post-marketing surveillance of drugs. We are here to ensure that FDA has taken the necessary actions to ensure better communication between the Office of New Drugs and the Office of Drug Safety and that the public is informed regarding the safety of drugs. Finally, we are here to examine Merck's responsibility in informing physicians and the public about the efficacy and safety of Vioxx.

Mr. WAXMAN. Thank you, Chairman Davis, for holding this hearing today.

I also want to thank you and your staff for leading this investigation into drug safety in the United States. You have asked tough questions and requested the information that the committee needs to have to perform its essential oversight function.

On the subject of Vioxx, there are many tough questions. Today's hearing focuses on one of the most important: why did so many doctors prescribe Vioxx for so long? Vioxx was approved in May 1999. Less than a year later, Merck announced at a major clinical trial, Vioxx was associated with four to five times more heart attack than naproxen, another anti-inflammatory drug.

Over the next year and a half, additional concerns were raised by an FDA advisory committee, by articles in the New York Times, and by the Journal of the American Medical Association. Yet sales continued to surge. Vioxx reached $2 billion in sales faster than any other drug in Merck's history. At the time of its withdrawal, after the cardiovascular risks were confirmed in another major study, over 100 million Vioxx prescriptions in the United States had been filled.

We now know that many of these prescriptions were dangerous and unnecessary. Over-prescription of a dangerous drug can be a public health disaster. In the case of Vioxx, experts have estimated that as many as 140,000 Americans may have suffered unnecessary heart attacks and strokes and other serious medical complications from the drug. It is critical to understand what went wrong; why did doctors write so many Vioxx prescriptions, even as evidence of harm mounted.

An important issue is whether FDA reacted too slowly to evidence of Vioxx's danger. It took FDA over 2 years to add a discussion of cardiovascular risks to Vioxx's label. FDA took nearly 3 years to conduct its own epidemiological of Vioxx safety. The agency never forced Merck to conduct a study specifically to address cardiovascular safety.

My conclusion is that FDA should have done more to understand the risks and protect the public. The question we all need to ask is how can we prevent this from happening in the future. Congress needs to give the agency new authorities and additional resources to ensure the safety of drugs after they are approved and marketed.

Today we will also discuss Merck's actions. Let me start by saying that Merck deserves credit for conducting important research on Vioxx safety, presenting this research at major medical meetings and publishing the studies in leading medical journals. But a company's responsibility does not end with publishing its research. What Merck said about its research findings to doctors and consumers and what Merck failed to say has critical importance.

One part of this equation is well-known, Merck's direct to consumer advertising. Merck spent over $300 million on consumer advertisements for Vioxx. Probably everyone in this room saw Dorothy Hamill on television skating in circles because of Vioxx, and certainly on behalf of Vioxx. Today we will focus on the hidden side of pharmaceutical promotion, how Merck communicated about Vioxx to physicians.

Merck employed more than 3,000 sales representatives to promote Vioxx to doctors and hospitals. These Merck representatives were extraordinarily well trained. Our committee has examined more than 20,000 pages of documents. These documents show that Merck trained their sales force to explore virtually every interaction with physicians. Merck and the drug industry say that the role of drug representatives is to educate doctors about new products, about new medical research.

But the documents tell a very different story. The goal was sales, not education. Merck representatives were instructed to use subtle gestures subconsciously to gain the trust of physicians. They were permitted to discuss only approved Journal articles, defined by Merck as articles that "provide solid evidence as to why doctors should prescribe Merck products" and health risks reviewed as "obstacles" that the sales force was instructed to surmount.

The first evidence of Vioxx's health risks was disclosed in March 2000, when Merck published the VIGOR study. VIGOR is going to be referred to a number of times, so let me say it is the Vioxx Gastrointestinal Outcomes Research [VIGOR]. This was announced to the public on March 27, 2000. This study showed that Vioxx had five times greater cardiovascular risks than naproxen.

Doctors naturally asked Merck's representatives about the implications of this Merck study. In response, Merck gave its representatives a cardiovascular card that indicated that Vioxx was actually 8 to 11 times safer than anti-inflammatory drugs like naproxen. I have a blow-up of that card, although obviously they had a smaller one. So we'll look at the total mortality. Vioxx 0.1, NSAIDs, meaning other anti-inflammatory drugs, 1.1, cardiovascular mortality, 0.1 as compared to 0.8. This card was shown over and over by these drug representatives to answer the question by telling people, doctors, that they should not worry about the mortality of using Vioxx.

Well, as we know now, this cardiovascular card was inaccurate and misleading. The data it cited did not support Merck's conclusions. During a staff briefing earlier this week by an FDA official, we were told that the relevance of the studies presented in the card to the cardiovascular safety of Vioxx was non-existent. According to the official, it would be ridiculous and scientifically inappropriate to use the data in the way Merck did.

Eleven months after the VIGOR study, an FDA advisory committee met to consider the study's implication. The committee concluded that doctors should be advised about the risks that Merck had found. But they were not advising doctors about it.

But here is how Merck responded. The very day after the FDA advisory committee said that doctors should be informed about the VIGOR study, Merck sent a bulletin to its sales representatives that stated, "Do not initiate discussions on the FDA advisory committee or the results of the VIGOR study." The same thing happened in May 2001 after a New York Times expose highlighted the dangers of Vioxx. Merck sent a bulletin to its field representatives that stated, "Do not initiate discussions on the results of the VIGOR study or any of the recent articles in the press on Vioxx."

Instead of informing doctors about the risks of Vioxx, Merck told its representatives to continue to rely on the highly questionable cardiovascular card. In fact, Merck gave its sales force a specific script to use with doctors when showing them the card, telling them to say to doctors that cardiovascular mortality of Vioxx was eight times lower than other drugs.

A few months later, JAMA published a critical article about Vioxx safety risks. Merck's response was to launch "Project Offense" to overcome the cardiovascular obstacle. Its sales team was told to quickly and effectively address all physician obstacles and return to the core message for Vioxx. The Merck documents are complex and the details are important, so my staff prepared a detailed briefing memo that summarizes the key documents and places them in perspective. I will make this document available to members and to witnesses.

When I step back and look at the big picture, here's what I see. Merck says the mission of its 3,000 person sales force is to educate doctors. And by the way, they spend more money on the sales force than they do on the direct to consumer advertising. This sales force is given extraordinary training so that it can capitalize on virtually every interaction with a doctor. Yet when it comes to the one thing the doctors most needed to know about Vioxx, its health risks, Merck's answer seems to be disinformation and censorship.

Merck's sales representatives were trained to see as if lives depended on it, but ultimately, their message may have cost lives instead. This is not an easy hearing for me. I have worked with Merck for decades. I know that Merck usually has high standards for corporate conduct and has produced many life-saving drugs.

But the purpose of oversight is to ask hard questions. The case of Vioxx reveals a side of pharmaceutical marketing that is rarely exposed. It is essential for the public, medical professionals and FDA to be aware of what happened here, so that we can prevent unnecessary injuries to patients in the future.

I thank the witnesses for coming and I look forward to their testimony today.

[The prepared statement of Hon. Henry A. Waxman follows:]

**Statement of Rep. Henry A. Waxman
For the Hearing, "The Roles of FDA and Pharmaceutical Companies in
Ensuring the Safety of Approved Drugs, Like Vioxx."**

May 5, 2005

Thank you, Chairman Davis, for holding this hearing today. I also would like to thank you and your staff for leading this investigation into drug safety in the United States. You have asked tough questions and requested the information that the Committee needs to perform its essential oversight function.

On the subject of Vioxx, there are many tough questions. Today's hearing focuses on one of the most important: Why did so many doctors prescribe so much Vioxx for so long?

Vioxx was approved in May 1999. Less than a year later, Merck announced that in a major clinical trial, Vioxx was associated with four to five times more heart attacks than naproxen, another anti-inflammatory drug. Over the next year and half, additional concerns were raised by an FDA advisory committee and by articles in the *New York Times* and the *Journal of the American Medical Association*.

Yet sales continued to surge. Vioxx reached $2 billion in sales faster than any drug in Merck's history. At the time of its withdrawal, after the cardiovascular risks were confirmed in another major study, over 100 million Vioxx prescriptions in the United States had been filled.

We now know that many of these prescriptions were dangerous and unnecessary.

Overprescription of a dangerous drug can be a public health disaster. In the case of Vioxx, experts have estimated that as many as 140,000 Americans may have suffered unnecessary heart attacks, strokes, and other serious medical complications from the drug.

It is critical to understand what went wrong. Why did doctors write so many Vioxx prescriptions even as evidence of harm mounted?

An important issue is whether FDA reacted too slowly to evidence of Vioxx's dangers. It took FDA over two years to add a discussion of cardiovascular risks to the Vioxx label. FDA took nearly three years to conduct its own epidemiological study of Vioxx's safety. And the agency never forced Merck to conduct a study specifically to address cardiovascular safety.

My conclusion is that FDA should have done more to understand the risk and protect the public. The question we all need to ask is how we can prevent this from happening in the future. Congress needs to give the agency new authorities and additional resources to ensure the safety of drugs after they are approved and marketed.

Today, we will also discuss Merck's actions. Let me start by saying that Merck deserves credit for conducting important research on Vioxx's safety, presenting this research at major medical meetings, and publishing the studies in leading medical journals.

But a company's responsibility does not end with publishing its research. What Merck said about its research findings to doctors and consumers — and what Merck failed to say — has critical importance.

One part of this equation is well known: Merck's direct-to-consumer advertisements. Merck spent over $300 million dollars on consumer advertisements for Vioxx. Probably everyone in this room saw Dorothy Hamill on television skating in circles on behalf of Vioxx.

Today, we will focus on the hidden side of pharmaceutical promotion: how Merck communicated about Vioxx to physicians.

Merck employed more than 3,000 sales representatives to promote Vioxx to doctors and hospitals. These Merck representatives were extraordinarily well trained. Our Committee has examined more than 20,000 pages of documents. These documents show that Merck trained their sales force to exploit virtually every interaction with physicians.

Merck and the drug industry say that the role of drug representatives is to educate doctors about new products and new medical research. But the documents tell a different story.

The goal was sales, not education. Merck representatives were instructed to use subtle gestures to subconsciously gain the trust of physicians. They were permitted to discuss only "approved" journal articles, defined by Merck as articles that "provide solid evidence as to why [doctors] should prescribe Merck products." And health risks were viewed as "obstacles" that the sales force was instructed to surmount.

The first evidence of Vioxx's health risks were disclosed in March 2000, when Merck published the VIGOR study. This study showed that Vioxx had five times greater cardiovascular risks than naproxen.

Doctors naturally asked Merck's representatives about the implications of Merck's study. In response, Merck gave its representatives a "Cardiovascular Card" that indicated that Vioxx was actually eight to eleven times <u>safer</u> than anti-inflammatory drugs like naproxen.

As we now know, this Cardiovascular Card was inaccurate and misleading. The data it cited did not support Merck's conclusions. During a staff briefing earlier this week, an FDA official said that the relevance of the studies presented in the card to the cardiovascular safety of Vioxx was "nonexistent." According to the official, it would be "ridiculous" and "scientifically inappropriate" to use the data in the way Merck did.

Eleven months after the VIGOR study, an FDA advisory committee met to consider the study's implications. The committee concluded that doctors should be advised about the risks that Merck had found.

But here's how Merck responded: the very day after the FDA advisory committee said that doctors should be informed about the VIGOR study, Merck sent a bulletin to its sales representatives that stated: "DO NOT INITIATE DISCUSSIONS ON THE FDA

ADVISORY COMMITTEE … OR THE RESULTS OF THE …VIGOR STUDY."

The same thing happened in May 2001 after a *New York Times* expose highlighted the dangers of Vioxx. Merck sent a bulletin to its field representatives that stated: "DO NOT INITIATE DISCUSSIONS ON THE RESULTS OF THE … VIGOR STUDY OR ANY OF THE RECENT ARTICLES IN THE PRESS ON VIOXX."

Instead of informing doctors about the risks of Vioxx, Merck told its representatives to continue to rely on the highly questionable Cardiovascular Card. In fact, Merck gave its sales force a specific script to use with doctors when showing them the card, telling them to say to doctors that the cardiovascular mortality of Vioxx was eight times lower than other drugs.

A few months later, *JAMA* published a critical article about Vioxx's safety risks. Merck's response was to launch "Project Offense" to overcome the cardiovascular "obstacle." Its sales team was told to "quickly and effectively address all physician obstacles and return to the core messages for VIOXX."

The Merck documents are complex and the details are important, so my staff prepared a detailed briefing memo that summarizes the key documents and places them in perspective. I will make this document available to members and the witnesses.

When I step back and look for the big picture, here's what I see. Merck says the mission of its 3,000-person sales force is to educate doctors. This sales force is given extraordinary training so that it can capitalize on virtually every interaction with doctors. Yet when it comes to the one thing doctors most needed to know about Vioxx — its health risks — Merck's answer seems to be disinformation and censorship.

Merck's sales representatives were trained to sell as if lives depended upon it. But ultimately, their message may have cost lives instead.

This is not an easy hearing for me. I have worked with Merck for decades, and I know that Merck usually has high standards for corporate conduct and has produced many life-saving drugs.

But the purpose of oversight is to ask the hard questions. And the case of Vioxx reveals a side of pharmaceutical marketing that is rarely exposed. It is essential for the public, medical professionals, and FDA to be aware of what happened here, so that we can prevent unnecessary injuries to patients in the future.

I thank the witnesses for coming and look forward to their testimony today.

Chairman TOM DAVIS. Thank you, and let me just add, Merck is here voluntarily to answer some of the issues that you have raised on this. I'm sure they will have a little bit different slant on it than you do. But we are here to get the facts and we appreciate everybody being with us.

Members will have 7 days to submit opening statements. I want to now recognize the first panel. We have Dr. Steven Galson, the Director of the Center for Drug Evaluation and Research of the Food and Drug Administration. He is accompanied by Dr. John Jenkins, the Director of the Office of New Drugs, the Center for Drug Evaluation and Research, and Dr. Paul Seligman, the Director of the Office of Pharmacoepidemiology in the Center for Drug Evaluation and Research, Food and Drug Administration and former Acting Director, Office of Drug Safety.

It is our policy that we swear our witnesses before you testify. Will you please rise with me and raise your right hands.

[Witnesses sworn.]

Chairman TOM DAVIS. Thank you very much for being here.

Dr. Galson, are you going to be the person who testifies and they are here for the questions? Is that how it's going to work?

Dr. GALSON. That's right.

Chairman TOM DAVIS. Thank you very much.

Yes, Mr. Waxman? We have documents we are putting into the record.

I would like to submit for the record all of the documents that are contained in the binders that have been provided to Members. If there is no objection, it will be so ordered. Thank you.

[NOTE.—The information referred to is on file with the committee.]

Chairman TOM DAVIS. Dr. Galson, thanks for being with us today.

STATEMENTS OF STEVEN GALSON, M.D., M.P.H., ACTING DIRECTOR, CENTER FOR DRUG EVALUATION AND RESEARCH, U.S. FOOD AND DRUG ADMINISTRATION, ACCOMPANIED BY JOHN JENKINS, DIRECTOR, OFFICE OF NEW DRUGS, CENTER FOR DRUG EVALUATION AND RESEARCH; AND PAUL SELIGMAN, DIRECTOR, OFFICE OF PHARMACOEPIDEMIOLOGY, CENTER FOR DRUG EVALUATION AND RESEARCH

Dr. GALSON. Mr. Chairman and members of the committee, I am Dr. Steven Galson, Acting Director of the Center for Drug Evaluation and Research at the Food and Drug Administration, and a Rear Admiral in the U.S. Public Health Service. Accompanying me today are Dr. John Jenkins, Director of the Office of New Drugs, and Dr. Paul Seligman, Director of our Office of Pharmacoepidemiology and Statistical Sciences, in which the Office of Drug Safety is located. He is also a captain in the U.S. Public Health Service.

I am pleased to be here today to discuss the relationship between the Center for Drug's Office of New Drugs and Office of Drug Safety as well as recent agency initiatives regarding drug safety. I would like to start by pointing out that the FDA's drug review process is recognized world-wide as the gold standard. We believe that FDA maintains the highest standards for drug approval and that drugs in the United States today are safer than they have ever been.

Why is this? FDA provides oversight at all stages of drug development. Early in this process, animal studies provide guidance on initial dosing and point to areas of safety needing special attention during human studies. Products usually undergo three phases of human clinical trials. Once the results of these trials are available, the sponsor analyzes the data and submits the new drug application or biologics license application to FDA.

FDA will only approve a drug after a sponsor demonstrates that its benefits outweigh its risks and that the drug meets the statutory standard for safety and efficacy. To make this determination, FDA reviewers conduct intensive analyses of all data submitted. At least half the effort of FDA's pre-market reviewers is dedicated to the assessment of safety.

Although we carry out a very thorough review and ask for a great deal of data, we recognize that there is no way we can anticipate all possible effects of the drug from the clinical trials that precede approval. After FDA approves a drug, the post-marketing monitoring stage begins. The role of our post-marketing safety system is to detect serious, unexpected adverse events and take definitive action when needed.

Sponsors are required to submit to FDA safety updates for seriously and previously unidentified risks in an expedited fashion and periodically for less urgent safety issues. These include reports of adverse events in which the company has been informed as well as new study results that have become available, whether or not they are published.

We also receive adverse events reports directly from health care providers and patients through our MedWatch program. All adverse events reports are stored in a common, computerized data base along with components of the periodic reports for selected drugs. FDA epidemiologists and safety evaluators review the reports and assess the frequency and seriousness of adverse events.

In addition, even after a drug is approved, FDA reviewers in the Office of New Drugs carefully examine the results of new clinical trials. It is worth noting that several of the most conspicuous recent safety issues, pediatric suicidality related to antidepressants and cardiovascular toxicity with the anti-inflammatory drugs, arose from randomized clinical trials conducted after approval or conducted with approved marketed products.

Decisions about regulatory action in response to evidence of a drug safety risk are complex. Our action will depend on the characteristics of the adverse event, the frequency of the reports, the seriousness of the diseases or conditions for which the drug provides a benefit, the availability of alternative therapy and the consequences of not treating the disease. Our Office of New Drugs and the Office of Drug Safety work very closely together in this process. New Drugs has authority for making decisions about whether a product will be approved for marketing.

At the time of reviewing a new drug application for marketing approval, however, they frequently engage with the Office of Drug Safety in discussing the overall safety profile of the drug and request their assistance in deciding what types of post-marketing studies should be requested. Once a drug is approved, post-marketing drug safety is a shared responsibility between both offices. There are times when post-marketing surveillance data alone cannot answer an important safety question about drugs. In such cases, the Office of Drug Safety can use its independent authority to pursue its own epidemiologic investigations.

Recent events related to the safety profile of the anti-inflammatory drugs are illustrative of the critical roles of both offices. On April 7, 2005, FDA issued a public health advisory to inform the public and health care community of a series of important changes pertaining to the marketing of these drugs. The Office of New Drugs and the Office of Drug Safety worked together and shared information and scientific analyses to reach consensus on these proposed changes. A close working relationship between these two offices was critical to the success of this action.

Let me quickly now describe some of the overall changes we are making in our safety program to respond to a lot of the concerns that we have heard. In November, Acting Commissioner Crawford announced a five-step plan to strengthen our drug safety program. It called for FDA to sponsor an Institute of Medicine study to evaluate the current drug safety system. In addition, we will implement a program for addressing differences of professional opinion, conduct a national search to fill the vacant position of the ODS director, conduct additional workshops and advisory committees to discuss complex drug safety and risk management issues and publish guidance that the agencies develop to help the pharmaceutical firms manage risks.

In addition to these steps, in February, HHS Secretary Leavitt and Acting Commissioner Crawford unveiled a new vision to promote a culture of transparency, openness and enhanced oversight within the agency, including the creation of a new Drug Safety Oversight Board to provide independent oversight and advice on the management of important drug safety issues and to manage the dissemination of certain safety information through our Web site.

We are pleased to report that today, FDA has posted two documents on its Web site to further our commitment to our drug safety initiative. The first of these going up today is a description of the organizational structure, role and responsibility of the Drug Safety Oversight Board. The second is that we have made available for comment a draft guidance entitled FDA's Drug Watch for Emerging Drug Safety Information. This document explains how FDA intends to develop and disseminate emerging drug safety information concerning marketed drug products to health care professionals and patients. The proposed drug watch Web page will post significant emerging safety information the FDA has received about certain drugs while the agency continues to actively evaluate the public health relevance of the information.

At FDA, providing the American public with safe and effective medical products is our core mission. We base decisions to improve a drug or to keep it on the market if new safety findings surface on a careful balancing of risk and benefit to patients. We will continue to evaluate new approaches to advance drug safety. As always, we value input from Congress, patients and the medical community.

Thank you very much for the opportunity to testify before you today. We are happy to respond to questions.

[The prepared statement of Dr. Galson follows:]

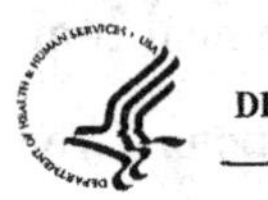

DEPARTMENT OF HEALTH & HUMAN SERVICES

Public Health Service

Food and Drug Administration
Rockville MD 20857

STATEMENT OF

STEVEN GALSON, M.D., M.P.H.

ACTING DIRECTOR

CENTER FOR DRUG EVALUATION AND RESEARCH

U.S. FOOD AND DRUG ADMINISTRATION

DEPARTMENT OF HEALTH AND HUMAN SERVICES

BEFORE THE

COMMITTEE ON
GOVERNMENT REFORM

UNITED STATES HOUSE OF REPRESENTATIVES

MAY 5, 2005

Release Only Upon Delivery

INTRODUCTION

Mr. Chairman and members of the Committee, I am Dr. Steven Galson, Acting Director of the Center for Drug Evaluation and Research (CDER), United States Food and Drug Administration (FDA or the Agency). I am pleased to be here today to discuss the relationship between CDER's Office of New Drugs (OND) and Office of Drug Safety (ODS) within the context of FDA's pre-market and post-market drug approval process, as well as recent Agency initiatives regarding drug safety.

SAFETY IS A HIGH PRIORITY

Modern drugs provide unmistakable and significant health benefits. FDA's drug review process is recognized worldwide as a gold standard. Indeed, we believe that FDA maintains the highest standards for drug approval. There have been significant additions to those standards during the last several decades, in response to advances in medical science. Currently, FDA approves drugs after they are studied in many more patients and undergo more detailed safety evaluations than ever before. It is not always recognized, but at least half of the effort of FDA's pre-market reviewers is dedicated to the assessment of safety. Major changes have taken place in how drugs are evaluated, including a complete evaluation of their metabolism, their interactions with other drugs, and potential differences of effectiveness or safety in people of different genders, ages, and races. In addition, internal guidance now describes an approach to the systematic assessment of safety that yields a comprehensive review, focusing on the potential problems with the greatest clinical importance.

FDA grants approval to drugs after a sponsor demonstrates that their benefits outweigh their risks for a specific population and a specific use, and that the drug meets the statutory standard for safety and efficacy. However, no amount of study before marketing will ever elucidate all the information about effectiveness or all the risks of a new drug. FDA recognizes that there is no way we can anticipate all possible effects of a drug from the clinical trials that precede approval. That is why Congress has supported and FDA has created a post-market drug safety program designed to collect and assess adverse events identified after approval. The role of our post-marketing safety system is to detect serious unexpected adverse events and take definitive action when needed.

FDA uses information from post-marketing clinical trials, adverse event reports filed by drug manufacturers, spontaneous reporting of adverse events by physicians, pharmacists, and consumers, and observational studies to identify problems in marketed products. FDA staff monitors this information and looks for emerging patterns. The Agency initiates action as needed.

THE DRUG APPROVAL PROCESS

<u>Pre-Approval Focus on Safety</u>

FDA's focus on safety begins at the earliest stages of drug development. Before beginning any human trials, the sponsor must perform extensive animal toxicity studies. Animal studies provide guidance on initial dosing and point to areas of safety needing special attention during human studies. Researchers closely monitor these studies and FDA reviews results in detail to be sure that giving the drug to humans is safe. FDA's oversight becomes more robust when human testing begins and we review a product under an investigational new drug application (IND). During the IND period, products usually undergo three phases of clinical (human) trials. Phase I studies involve the initial introduction of a drug into humans to assess the most common side effects and examine the range of doses that patients can take safely without a high rate of side effects.

Phase I studies also gain information on drug kinetics and metabolism, drug-drug interactions, and, often, on the effects of the drug on the electrocardiogram. Phase I trials may be in patients with the disease the experimental drug is being developed to treat, but also may be in healthy volunteer subjects. In general, these studies yield initial safety data and useful information to establish the appropriate dose of the drug.

Phase II of drug development includes the earliest controlled clinical studies of the effectiveness of the drug for a specific indication in patients with the disease or condition. This phase of testing also identifies short-term, relatively common side effects of the drug. Phase II studies are typically well controlled and closely monitored and may involve up to several hundred patients. In these studies, researchers compare results of patients receiving the drug with those who receive a placebo, a different dose of the test drug, and/or another active drug. At the conclusion of these studies, FDA and the sponsor usually meet to determine how the drug's development should be studied in Phase III and how to design and conduct further trials.

Researchers design Phase III trials for a larger number of patients and build on the data gained from the first two phases of trials. These studies provide the additional information about safety and effectiveness needed to evaluate the overall benefit-risk relationship of the drug. The larger number of patients (typically several thousand) allows detection of less frequent adverse events. The larger number of patients (typically 300-600) exposed for more than 6 months allows detection of adverse events that develop only after longer exposure. Phase III study designs establish the basis for extrapolating the results to the general population. It is results of these studies that usually provide essential information for the package labeling. Once the results of all the clinical trials are available, the sponsor of the application (usually the manufacturer of the product) analyzes all the data and submits a new drug application (NDA) or biologics license application (BLA) to FDA for review and approval to market the product in the U.S.

Pre-marketing assessment of the safety aspects of an application is critical to the determination of whether a drug can be approved and this assessment represents about half of the effort involved in a review, both in time spent and in documentation.
To assure a complete and consistent review of safety of an NDA or BLA, in February 2005, FDA issued a guidance to reviewers for conducting and preparing reports of clinical safety reviews. See *http://www.fda.gov/ohrms/dockets/ac/05/briefing/2005-4143B1_06_Tab-13.pdf*. This document is a collaborative effort across various offices in CDER, including OND and ODS. The guidance assists reviewers conducting the clinical NDA/BLA safety reviews, describes good review practices for pre-marketing safety reviews, provides standardization and consistency of format and content of safety reviews, and ensures that critical presentations and analyses of safety data are not omitted.

Post-Approval Risk Assessment

Once FDA approves a drug, the post-marketing monitoring stage begins. The sponsor (typically the manufacturer) is required to submit safety updates to FDA on their drug. These updates are submitted in an expedited fashion for serious and previously unidentified risks, and periodically for less urgent safety issues. These reports include reports of adverse events of which the company has been informed, as well as new study results that are available whether published or not (including those published in other countries). Also during this period, we continuously receive adverse event reports directly from sources such as health care providers and patients through our own MedWatch program. Expedited adverse event reports from sponsors or MedWatch are stored in a common computerized database along with components of the periodic reports for selected drugs. FDA epidemiologists and safety evaluators review and analyze the reports to assess the frequency and seriousness of the adverse events. Our response to information from this ongoing surveillance depends on an evaluation of the aggregate public health benefit of the product compared to its evolving risk profile.

Decisions about regulatory action in response to evidence of a drug safety risk are complex, taking into account many factors. The occurrence of a rare event, even a serious event, may or may not, by itself, be sufficient to take a drug product off the market. If the public health benefit of the product outweighs its known risks, FDA generally allows the continued marketing of the drug. Often, as more becomes known about the potential risks or benefits of a product, its label will be revised so that it better reflects information on appropriate use. For example, FDA may ask the manufacturer to revise the labeling to add information on adverse reactions not previously listed, to add new warnings describing conditions under which the drug should not be used, or to add new precautions advising doctors of measures to minimize risk. FDA often issues Public Health Advisories and information sheets for health care providers and patients that discuss the new safety information. In the event of reports of death or life-threatening injury, FDA and the sponsor may consider restricting the distribution of the product or removing it from the market.

Our action will depend on the characteristics of the adverse events, the frequency of the reports, the seriousness of the diseases or conditions for which the drug provides a benefit, the availability of alternative therapy, and the consequences of not treating the disease. Detection and limiting adverse reactions can be challenging. Weighing the impact of adverse drug reactions against the benefits of a particular product is multifaceted and complex, and involves scientific as well as public health issues.

Attachment A contains the sequence of events with Vioxx from the opening of the IND on December 20, 1994, until the public announcement of worldwide withdrawal on September 30, 2004, and also may be found on FDA's website at *http://www.fda.gov/ohrms/dockets/ac/05/briefing/2005-4090B1_04_E-FDA-TAB-C.htm*. This document demonstrates the give and take between the Agency and sponsors in negotiating labeling changes when adverse events occur that warrant Agency action.

Independent Offices in CDER Foster Critical Communication and Cooperation

A sound program for assessing the safety of drugs, particularly weighing risks against benefits, demands integrated expertise from a variety of disciplines and perspectives. In CDER, physicians, pharmacists, toxicologists, chemists, epidemiologists, statisticians, bio-pharmaceutics experts, and clinical pharmacologists share drug safety assessments. These experts work in many organizational components of the Center, but predominantly in OND and ODS. These offices work closely together, but are in different organizational components of the Center, thereby ensuring their reporting and operating independence. As in any scientific organization, the ability for scientists to develop independent perspectives on a given issue and bring consensus to decisions depends on strong communication at all working levels, leadership and a sense of shared responsibility.

Safety assessments in any given drug's life cycle begin in OND, where toxicologists and physicians review the animal data in support of Phase I studies, as well as each clinical study protocol and results of the studies in Phases I, II and III before a drug is marketed. Such assessments consider results of new animal studies beyond those that were used to justify initial clinical trials; reports of serious adverse events occurring in clinical studies that are submitted to FDA within days of their occurrence; results of studies of how a drug is metabolized once in the body; monitoring of the medical literature for current thinking about the drug as it may have been used in other countries, and many other sources of information. FDA staff conducts detailed reviews of all these sources and more before FDA approves a product for marketing. FDA will not approve a drug if its benefits in clinical trials are not thought to outweigh its risks as seen in the trial or if the clinical trials did not adequately assess safety.

There are times when a drug is approved, but CDER remains concerned that a particular aspect of its safety profile needs to be explored in more depth. These concerns might include, for example, a sub-population of patients who were not well represented in the pre-market studies, a question about how well the drug is tolerated in combination with other commonly prescribed drugs, or how the safety of the drug compares to a different drug to treat the same condition. In such cases, when we grant approval for marketing, we request a formal commitment from the sponsor to conduct such a study within a specified timeframe after approval.

CDER's OND has authority for making decisions about whether a product will be approved for marketing. OND is organized into 17 divisions that represent clinical areas of expertise, such as oncology, endocrinology, psychiatry and pulmonary medicine. Products are reviewed by the division that contains experts in the field of medicine that will primarily be the users of the product (e.g., asthma drugs would be reviewed by the division with pulmonary expertise). Pre-market safety assessments are often shared across divisions. When a drug being assessed in one division appears to have a side effect that might be better evaluated by a different type of clinical expert, an expert in another division will be consulted (e.g., an antibiotic might cause lung toxicity, so the pulmonary division would be consulted).

Also, at the time of reviewing an NDA for marketing approval, the OND review team routinely engages ODS in discussing the overall safety profile of the drug, and often requests their assistance in deciding what types of post-marketing studies should be requested of the company to address residual concerns. ODS' involvement in the review of a drug before marketing is particularly critical when the drug has a risk profile that warrants a complex risk management plan, such as a restricted distribution program or specialized educational tools for patients or health care providers about how best to use the drug.

Once a product is on the market, a sponsor may decide to study the drug for additional indications. In such a case, the application is in "pre-market" status regarding the new indication at the same time we are conducting post-market surveillance of the marketed product. This means that clinical study data, including adverse event reports from trials, will be submitted on a continuous basis and new studies for even more new indications or in new populations for the original indication may be started. All of these studies require review and monitoring by OND. At the same time, ODS continues to monitor the safety of the drug based on post-marketing adverse event reports that are submitted by companies or directly to FDA through the MedWatch program, all of which must be factored into decisions about design of the new studies and whether to approve new uses for the drug. ODS completes about 1300 safety reviews a year as well as participates in the development and review of over 40 risk management plans in close collaboration with OND.

When post-market surveillance data cannot answer an important safety question about a drug or group of drugs, ODS has independent authority to pursue its own epidemiology research. This independent research is highly valued in the scientific community when it conforms to accepted scientific standards and procedures such as sound scientific oversight and peer review. Research conducted by ODS epidemiologists employs a program of cooperative agreement mechanisms and contracts that allow FDA to have access to databases about drug usage and effects and to partner with non-government researchers to do the studies.

Factoring identified risks, whether from clinical trials, adverse event reports or epidemiology studies into the risk-benefit equation for a drug requires cooperation between OND and ODS. Each office offers expertise in evaluating the risk-benefit profiles of marketed drugs. OND is equipped to evaluate the NDA, including the clinical trial data, labeling information, and post-marketing studies. ODS brings unparalleled ability to identify emerging risks in new patient populations that may not have been seen during pre-market clinical trials. It is only through the contributions of these two offices that the most accurate assessment of a drug's risk-benefit profile can be made.

The Agency believes CDER's current organizational structure has significant benefits. Having both independent offices in FDA's CDER ensures efficient decision-making, expeditious resolution of disputes and the rapid dissemination of critical drug safety information to the public and health care providers.

Turning Risk-Assessment into Action—Joint Efforts of OND and ODS

Recent events related to the safety profile of non-steroidal anti-inflammatory drugs are illustrative of the critical roles of both OND and ODS in arriving at sound scientific decisions and public health policy on regulatory actions for drugs.

On April 7, 2005, FDA issued a Public Health Advisory to inform the public and health care community of a series of important changes pertaining to the marketing of the non-steroidal anti-inflammatory class of drugs (NSAIDs), including COX-2 selective and prescription and non-prescription (over-the-counter (OTC)) non-selective NSAID medications. After carefully considering the available data on all of the NSAIDs, including the presentations, discussions, and votes from the joint public meeting of the FDA Arthritis Advisory Committee and the Drug Safety and Risk Management Advisory Committee held on February 16, 17, and 18, 2005, FDA took action to immediately address the cardiovascular (CV) safety concerns for these drugs along with their overall risk-benefit profile. FDA's actions are summarized, as follows:

> 1. FDA asked Pfizer, Inc. to voluntarily withdraw Bextra (valdecoxib) from the market. Pfizer has agreed to suspend sales and marketing of Bextra in the U.S., pending further discussions with the Agency.
>
> 2. FDA asked manufacturers of all marketed prescription NSAIDs, including Celebrex, (celecoxib), a COX-2 selective NSAID, to revise the labeling (package insert) for their products to include a boxed warning and a Medication Guide. The boxed warning will highlight the potential for increased risk of CV events with these drugs and the well described, serious, and potentially life-threatening gastrointestinal (GI) bleeding associated with their use. The Medication Guide will accompany every prescription NSAID at the time it is dispensed to better inform patients about the CV and GI risks.
>
> 3. FDA asked manufacturers of non-prescription NSAIDs to revise their labeling to include more specific information about the potential GI and CV risks, and information to assist consumers in the safe use of the drug. This announcement

does not apply to aspirin as it has clearly been shown to reduce the risk of serious adverse CV events in certain patient populations.

It was only through shared information and consensus across OND and ODS that these actions were decided.   Several examples of this are as follows:

- OND and ODS jointly made the determination that the lack of adequate data on the CV safety of long-term use of Bextra, along with the increased risk of adverse CV events in clinical studies of short-term coronary artery bypass surgery (CABG) suggested that the risk of Bextra was probably relevant to chronic use.

- ODS analyzed post-marketing reports of serious and potentially life-threatening skin reactions, including deaths, in patients using Bextra. The ODS and OND reviews of the reports of these reactions in individual patients led to the consensus that the reaction is unpredictable, occurring in patients with and without a prior history of sulfa allergy, and after both short- and long-term use.

- OND's reconsideration of the original NDA data for Bextra confirmed the lack of any demonstrated advantages for Bextra compared with other NSAIDs.

- It was through much discussion across OND and ODS, including consideration of the advice from two Advisory Committees, that led CDER to conclude that the benefits of Celebrex outweigh the potential risks in properly selected and informed patients. Accordingly, FDA will allow Celebrex to remain on the market as long as a box warning about the GI and CV risks of the drug are implemented.

- It required the different perspectives from OND and ODS, evaluating multiple sources of data, for CDER to conclude that both CV and GI adverse events are likely to be common to the entire class of NSAIDS, new and old (with the exception of CV risk for
low-dose aspirin). The importance of the different types of expertise that facilitated that decision-making (clinical trial design and analysis, statistics, clinical pharmacology, pharmacovigilance, epidemiology and clinical medicine) cannot be overemphasized.

The April 6, 2005, summary memorandum, "Analysis and recommendations for Agency action regarding non-steroidal anti-inflammatory drugs and cardiovascular risks," co-signed by John Jenkins, M.D., Director, OND, and Paul Seligman, M.D., Director, Office of Pharmacoepidemiology and Statistical Science (the organizational through which ODS reports) illustrates the close cooperation between the two offices. See Attachment B. This memo also may be found on FDA's website at: *www.fda.gov/cder/drug/infopage/COX2/NSAIDdecisionMemo.pdf.*

STATUTORY CHANGES ENHANCE DRUG APPROVAL AT FDA

FDA was founded in response to concerns about safety. Attention to safety pervades everything that we do. In the Federal Food, Drug and Cosmetic (FD&C) Act of 1938, Congress gave FDA the authority to review the evidence that a drug was safe for its intended use. In 1962, Congress added a requirement that drug sponsors also demonstrate that a drug is effective, using adequate and well-controlled studies. Thus, drug safety means that the demonstrated benefits of a drug outweigh its known and potential risks for the intended population and use. In recent years, Congress has enacted legislation that provides significant additional tools to improve our focus on safety: the Prescription Drug User Fee Act (PDUFA) and the Food and Drug Administration Modernization Act (FDAMA).

In 1992, Congress enacted PDUFA. This landmark legislation provided significant resources for FDA to hire more medical and scientific reviewers to conduct pre-market reviews, to hire support personnel and field investigators to speed the application review process for human drug and biological products, and to acquire critical information technology infrastructure to support our review process.

In 1997, following the success of PDUFA I, Congress reauthorized the program for an additional five years when it enacted FDAMA. With PDUFA II came additional goals designed to reduce drug development times. In 2002, Congress reauthorized PDUFA for a third time. PDUFA III places great emphasis on ensuring that user fees provide a sound financial footing for FDA's new drug and biologic review process and, for the first time, gives FDA authority to expend PDUFA resources on risk management and drug safety activities during the approval process and during the first two to three years following drug approval.

One of the primary goals of PDUFA was to address the significant delay in U.S. patients' access to new medicines. The objective was to increase patient access to new drugs, without increasing risks. Before PDUFA, the delay in approving drugs in the U.S. was a serious concern for U.S. patients and practitioners. Life-saving drugs were available to patients in other countries months and sometimes years before they were available in the U.S. Because of the additional resources and process improvements implemented since PDUFA I became law, the average FDA drug review time has declined by more than 12 months. While PDUFA gave FDA the resources needed to bring safe and effective drugs to the market faster, it did not change the high standards FDA employs in the review of NDAs. In fact, FDA's review standards remain the gold standard in the world.

A recent study by Berndt, et al. of the National Bureau of Economic Research, found no significant differences in the rates of safety withdrawals for drugs approved before PDUFA compared to drugs approved during the PDUFA era. This research confirms FDA's analysis on the same subject. In addition, as the public has become more aware of drug safety issues, we are now adding box warnings sooner than we did before PDUFA. This indicates that PDUFA has been successful in both speeding access and preserving safety.

In general, PDUFA authorizes FDA to collect fees from companies that produce certain human drug and biological products. When a sponsor seeks FDA approval for a new drug or biologic product, it must submit an application accompanied by a fee to support the review process. In addition, companies pay annual fees for each manufacturing establishment and for each prescription drug product marketed. Before PDUFA, taxpayers alone paid for product reviews through budgets provided by Congress. Under the PDUFA approach, industry provides

additional funding in return for FDA's efforts to meet drug-review performance goals that emphasize timeliness but do not alter or compromise our commitment to ensuring that drugs are safe and effective before they are approved for marketing.

PDUFA III – GREATER EMPHASIS ON DRUG SAFETY

As noted above, thanks to PDUFA, we are able to commit far greater resources to our important safety responsibilities. Under PDUFA III, Congress granted authority for FDA to expend user fees for post-market safety review. FDA made this a top priority during our PDUFA negotiations. Beginning with PDUFA III, for drugs approved after October 1, 2002, we can spend PDUFA resources on "collecting, developing, and reviewing safety information on drugs, including adverse event reports" for up to three years after the date of approval. The initiative to address drug safety for PDUFA III products helps FDA better understand a drug's risk profile, provide risk feedback to the sponsors and provide essential safety information to patients and health practitioners.

From October 1, 2002, through December 31, 2004, FDA reviewed 63 risk management plans for drug and biologic products. Twenty-eight of these related to applications submitted after PDUFA III took effect. We also conducted pre-approval safety conferences, risk management plan reviews, drug safety meetings, and meetings with sponsors to discuss proposed drug supplements.

In response to PDUFA III, FDA held a public meeting in April 2003 to discuss risk assessment, risk management, and pharmacovigilance practices. On May 5, 2004, based on the valuable information generated through the meeting process, we published three draft guidances on these important drug safety topics. Following our review of the extensive comments we received about these documents, all three final guidances were published in April 2005.

SAFETY ADVANCES IN FDAMA

Enacted in 1997, FDAMA has been an important addition to FDA's legal framework. FDAMA passed following a thorough Congressional examination of the Agency's policies and programs. It instituted a number of comprehensive changes, reaffirmed the Agency's vital role in protecting the public health and served as the vehicle for enacting PDUFA II.

Pediatric Exclusivity and Safer Use of Drugs in Children

For decades, children were prescribed medications that had not been studied for safety and efficacy in pediatric populations. As a component of FDAMA, Congress provided incentives to sponsors to conduct pediatric clinical trials. Section 111 of FDAMA authorized FDA to grant an additional six months of marketing exclusivity (known as pediatric exclusivity) to pharmaceutical manufacturers that conduct studies of certain drugs in pediatric populations. The objective of section 111 was to promote pediatric safety and efficacy studies of drugs. With the valuable information generated by these studies, the product labeling can then be updated to include appropriate information on use of the drug in the pediatric population. To qualify for pediatric exclusivity, sponsors must conduct pediatric studies according to the terms of a Written Request issued by FDA and submit the results of those studies in an NDA or supplement.

In 2002, Congress renewed this authority when it enacted the Best Pharmaceuticals for Children Act (BPCA). BPCA also mandates that during the one-year period beginning on the date a drug receives exclusivity, FDA review and refer to the Pediatric Advisory Committee, in a public forum, any adverse event reports associated with the use of the drug. To date, we have referred to the Pediatric Advisory Committee at six separate meetings adverse event reports on 34 drugs.

Finally, BPCA contains important, new disclosure requirements. Outside of BPCA, the Agency generally may not publicly disclose information contained in an IND, unapproved NDA, or unapproved supplemental NDA. Once FDA approves an NDA or supplemental NDA, the Agency can make public certain summary information regarding the safety and effectiveness of the product for the approved indication.

However, section 9 of BPCA gives FDA important new disclosure authority. BPCA requires that, no later than 180 days after the submission of a supplement containing studies conducted in response to a Written Request, the Agency must publish a summary of FDA's medical and clinical pharmacology reviews of those studies. Moreover, we must publish this information regardless of whether our action on the pediatric supplement is an approval, approvable, or not-approvable action. Thus under FDAMA, information on pediatric studies conducted in response to Written Requests was not available until after the supplemental application was approved. In contrast, under BPCA, a summary of FDA's medical and clinical pharmacology reviews of pediatric studies is publicly available regardless of the action taken on the supplemental application. Since 2002, FDA has posted the summaries of these reviews for 41 products submitted in response to a Written Request on FDA's website at: *http://www.fda.gov/cder/pediatric/Summaryreview.htm.* This information provides a rich source of valuable safety information to allow pediatricians to make more informed decisions about whether and how to use these drugs in their patients.

Post-Marketing Safety Studies

On April 30, 2001, FDA's regulations implementing section 130 of FDAMA, which requires sponsors of approved drugs and biologics to report annually on the status of post-marketing commitments, became effective. These regulations modified existing reporting requirements for NDA drug studies and created a new reporting requirement for biologic products.

FDA may request that a sponsor conduct post-marketing studies to provide additional important information on how a drug works in expanded patient populations or to identify safety issues that occur at very low frequency or in special patient populations. Patient and consumer advocates who track the completion of post-marketing commitments and FDA's efforts to review study results and modify drug labeling are keenly interested in the post-marketing safety study reporting obligations in section 130. The regulations implementing section 130 provide FDA with a mechanism to monitor study progress through the annual submission of study status reports. FDA posts the status of post-marketing studies on its public website and publishes an annual summary of industry's progress in fulfilling post-marketing commitments in the *Federal Register*.

CRITICAL PATH

On March 16, 2004, FDA released a report addressing the recent slowdown in innovative medical therapies submitted to FDA for approval: "Innovation/Stagnation: Challenge and Opportunity on the Critical Path to New Medical Products." See, *http://www.fda.gov/oc/initiatives/criticalpath/whitepaper.html*. The report describes options to modernize the medical product development process to try to make it more predictable and less costly. The report focuses on ways that FDA could collaborate with academic researchers, product developers, patient groups, and other stakeholders to make the critical path much faster, predictable, and less costly. Improved safety tools and tools to help individualize therapy are integral parts of the Critical Path.

Enhancing the Safety of Medical Products

During drug development, safety issues should be detected as early as possible. However, because of limitations of current methods, safety problems are often uncovered only during clinical trials or, occasionally, after marketing. Some tools used for toxicology and human safety testing are outdated despite efforts to develop better methods. Clinical testing, even if extensive, often fails to detect important safety problems, either because they are uncommon or because the tested population was not representative of eventual recipients. Conversely, some models create worrisome signals that may not be predictive of a human safety problem.

There are opportunities for developing tools that can more reliably and efficiently determine the safety of a new medical product. To meet this challenge, FDA has called for a new focus on modernizing the tools that applied biomedical researchers and product developers use to assess the safety and effectiveness of potential new products. Many of these tools—diagnostics such as pharmacogenomic tests and imaging techniques—would also be used after marketing to monitor safety in the real world clinical setting. The Critical Path report describes opportunities for FDA, working with academia, patient groups, industry, and other government agencies, to embark on a collaborative research effort. The goal is to create new performance standards and predictive tools that will provide better answers about the safety and effectiveness of investigational products, to do this faster and with more certainty, and to enhance the safety of these products in the clinic.

In addition to improved safety tools, Critical Path also focuses on tools that will help individualize therapy. We enhance safety when the target population does not include individuals who cannot benefit from the treatment. For these individuals, drug exposure is all risk. Better tools for individualized therapy will help to identify patients who will respond to therapy and, very importantly, keep those who are at high risk for serious side effects from receiving the therapy. New science has provided the basic knowledge to make these tools a reality.

Critical Path is not a fundamental departure for FDA, but rather builds on the Agency's proven "best practices" for expediting the availability of promising medical technologies. While the report touches on all aspects of medical product development, identifying new tools to address drug safety challenges would represent a giant step down the Critical Path.

NEW FDA INITIATIVES TO STRENGTHEN DRUG SAFETY

<u>November 2004 Five-Step Plan</u>

At FDA, we are constantly striving to improve our processes and methods, and thereby better serve the public health. Recent developments have prompted us to refocus our drug safety efforts and take additional steps to identify drugs that may have unacceptable risk profiles.

On November 5, 2004, Acting FDA Commissioner Lester Crawford announced a five-step plan to strengthen FDA's drug safety program. First, it called for FDA to sponsor an IOM study to evaluate the current drug safety system. An IOM committee will study the effectiveness of the U.S. drug safety system, with an emphasis on the post-marketing phase, and assess what additional steps FDA could take to learn more about the side effects of drugs as they are actually used. We have asked IOM to examine FDA's role within the health care delivery system and recommend measures to enhance the confidence of Americans in the safety and effectiveness of their drugs. In recent weeks, the IOM announced the names of the experts who will conduct the study. We are confident that this distinguished panel will provide a thorough review of the drug safety system in this country and advise FDA on how to help ensure that drug safety assessments keep pace with other aspects of drug development.

Second, Dr. Crawford announced that CDER would implement a program for addressing differences of professional opinion. I am pleased to report that CDER has put this program into effect. In most cases, free and open discussion of scientific issues among review teams and with supervisors, managers and external advisors, leads to an agreed course of action. Sometimes, however, a consensus decision cannot be reached, and an employee may feel that his or her opinion was not adequately considered. In an effort to improve the current process, CDER has formalized a program to help ensure that the opinions of dissenting scientific reviewers are formally addressed and that FDA's decision-making process is transparent. An ad hoc panel, including FDA staff and outside experts not directly involved in disputed decisions, will have 30 days to review all relevant materials and recommend to the Center Director an appropriate course of action.

Third, CDER is conducting a national search to fill the currently vacant position of Director of the Office of Drug Safety, which is responsible for overseeing the post-marketing safety program for all drugs. CDER is seeking a candidate who is a nationally recognized drug safety expert with knowledge of the basic science of drug development and post-marketing surveillance, and a strong commitment to protecting the public health. CDER is working with the Office of Personnel Management on this search.

Fourth, in the coming year CDER will conduct additional workshops and advisory committee meetings to discuss complex drug safety and risk management issues. Most recently, for example, the Agency conducted a three-day Advisory Committee meeting that examined COX-2 selective NSAID drugs and related medicines. This meeting was held on February 16-18, 2005, and more than twenty-five experts made presentations. At the end of the meeting, the Advisory Committee issued recommendations that the Agency promptly and carefully reviewed before announcing a proposed regulatory action discussed below.

Finally, as promised by Dr. Crawford in his November announcement, FDA has now published final versions of three guidances that the Agency developed to help pharmaceutical firms manage risks involving drugs and biological products. These guidances will assist pharmaceutical firms in identifying and assessing potential safety risks before and after a drug reaches the market.

<u>February 2005 Drug Safety Announcement</u>

On February 15, 2005, Health and Human Services (HHS) Secretary Michael Leavitt and Acting FDA Commissioner Crawford unveiled a new, emboldened vision for FDA that will promote a culture of transparency, openness, and enhanced oversight within the Agency. As part of this vision, FDA plans to create a new Drug Safety Oversight Board (DSB) to provide independent oversight and advice on the management of important drug safety issues and to manage the dissemination of certain safety information through FDA's website to health care professionals and patients.

Under this proposal, FDA plans to enhance the independence of internal deliberations and decisions regarding risk/benefit analyses and consumer safety. The DSB will oversee the management of important drug safety issues within CDER. The DSB will include individuals from FDA, as well as medical experts from other HHS agencies and government departments (e.g., the National Institutes of Health and Department of Veterans Affairs). Individuals on the Board who have conducted the primary review of data or served as deciding officials for any regulatory action under consideration will be recused from voting on issues concerning those particular drugs. CDER's Deputy Director will serve as the Chair of the DSB. The DSB also will consult with other medical experts and representatives of patient and consumer groups. CDER is updating its Manuel of Policies and Procedures (MAPP) to reflect the organizational structure, roles, and responsibilities of DSB in CDER. Among other responsibilities described in the MAPP, the DSB and its staff will:

- Identify, track, and oversee the management of important drug safety issues;
- Adjudicate organizational disputes concerning the management of drug safety issues;
- Establish policies regarding management of drug safety issues in CDER;
- Select drugs to be placed on Drug Watch (described below) and update their status (including deciding to remove drugs from Drug Watch) as appropriate;
- Oversee the development of patient and professional information sheets in CDER;
- Track important emerging safety issues and ensure that they are resolved in a timely manner; and
- Ensure that CDER decisions about a drug's safety benefit from the input and perspective of experts within and outside FDA who have not conducted the primary review or served as a deciding official in the ongoing pre-market evaluation or post-market surveillance activities with respect to that drug.

FDA also plans to increase the transparency of the Agency's decision-making process by establishing new and expanding existing communication channels to provide drug safety information to the public. These communications will help ensure that established and emerging drug safety data are quickly available in an easily accessible form. The increased openness will enable patients and their health care professionals to make better-informed decisions about individual treatment options.

One communication mechanism the Agency is proposing is a new *Drug Watch* web page that will include emerging information about possible serious side effects or other safety risks for previously and newly approved drugs. This resource will contain valuable information that may affect patient selection or monitoring decisions. The web resource may also contain information about measures that patients and practitioners can take to prevent or mitigate harm. This information resource will significantly enhance public knowledge and understanding of safety issues by discussing emerging or potential safety problems, sometimes even before FDA has reached a conclusion that would prompt a regulatory action.

We are also intensifying our current efforts to provide the public with the most important information for the safe and effective use of drugs in patient-friendly language. We are doing this through the development of two tools: *Patient Information Sheets* and *Healthcare Professional Information Sheets*.

1. *Patient Information Sheets* are intended to convey critical facets of a product's approved labeling in lay terms. These sheets will also include a section for "emerging safety information" in those instances when we determine that there is information on the *Drug Watch* that a patient should consider. This "emerging safety information" will match the information on the *Drug Watch*. Information from the *Drug Watch* that is not in the final labeling of the product will be clearly

identifiable and accompanied by a disclaimer, such as: *"This information reflects FDA's preliminary analysis of data concerning this drug. FDA is considering, but has not reached a final conclusion about, this information. FDA intends to update this sheet when additional information or analyses become available."* Our ultimate objective is to develop Patient Information Sheets for all approved drugs, most of which will not have an emerging safety section.

2. *Healthcare Professional Information Sheets* are intended to highlight the most up-to-date information practitioners may want to consider in prescribing drugs for their patients. We ultimately intend to develop these sheets for all new molecular entities as well as some other drugs. This is not a new approach. When available, the highlights section of a product's approved labeling will be used to develop the *Healthcare Professional Information* sheets.

We have already posted some patient and *Healthcare Professional Information* sheets on our website for drugs with recent emerging safety issues. See for example, Celebrex patient and professional sheets, *http://www.fda.gov/cder/drug/infopage/celebrex/Celebrex-ptsk.pdf* and *http://www.fda.gov/cder/drug/infopage/celebrex/celebrex-hcp.pdf*. We intend to link the information that is on *Drug Watch* to patient and *Healthcare Professional Information* sheets when they are available.

As FDA develops these communication tools, the Agency will solicit public input on how FDA should manage potential concerns associated with disseminating emerging information prior to regulatory action. In addition, FDA will actively seek feedback from health care professionals, patients and consumers on how best to make this information available and useful to them.

Increased Funding for the Office of Drug Safety (ODS)

FDA has a longstanding commitment to drug safety. CDER devotes more than 50 percent of its current resources to critical regulatory activities to ensure drug safety throughout the entire life cycle of U.S. pharmaceuticals. Drug safety analysis is a collaborative effort by various offices across CDER. ODS is one such office involved in the overall drug safety function, with a primary focus on the evaluation of drug safety post-marketing. The graph, set forth below, demonstrates the steady increase in ODS' financial and human resources over the past decade.

The budget for fiscal year 2006 continues this commitment. The President has proposed a 24 percent increase for FDA's post-market safety program to help further ensure that America's pharmaceutical supply is safe and effective, and of the highest quality. Under this proposal, ODS would receive increased funding to expand the Agency's ability to rapidly survey, identify and respond to potential safety concerns for drugs on the market. ODS will hire additional staff to manage and lead safety reviews, will increase the number of staff with expertise in critical areas such as risk management, risk communication and epidemiology, and will increase access to a wide range of clinical, pharmacy and administrative databases. The Administration's proposed budget for ODS will increase by $6.5 million, including $1.5 million in user fees, for a total fiscal year 2006 ODS funding level of $33.4 million. PDUFA resources will represent nearly one-third of the ODS budget for the coming year. Our commitment to increase resources available for post-market safety will enhance the structural changes we are proposing to advance drug safety.

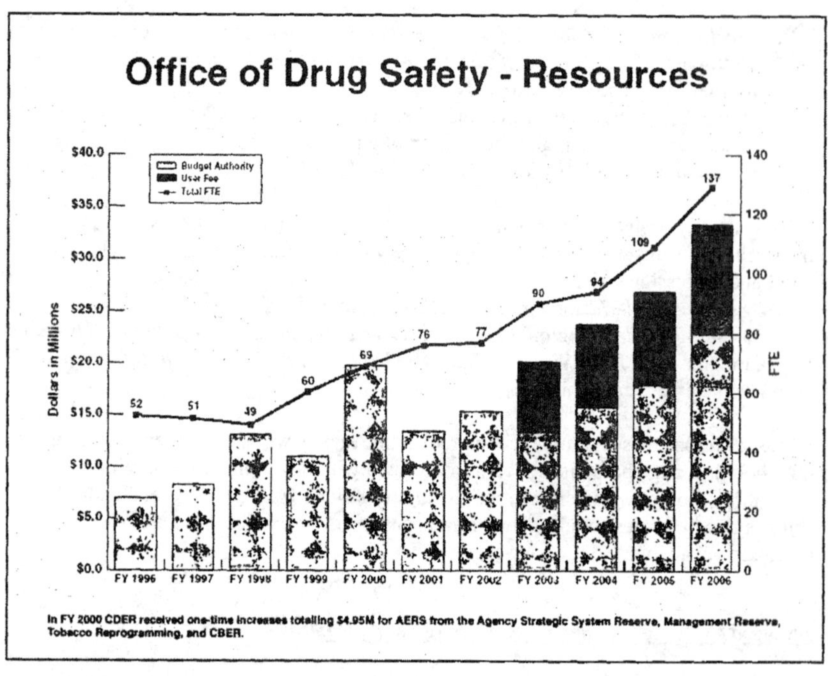

With the additional funds, FDA expects to be able to hire eight additional Full Time Equivalents (FTEs) in ODS to establish policies and processes regarding safety reviews and risk management, to manage communications with OND and to support patient safety initiatives and external partnerships with CMS, AHRQ, and other HHS Agencies.

We also plan to hire an additional 14 FTEs in the three operating divisions of ODS. These employees will handle the increased workload of monitoring biologic therapeutics; promote increased communication and coordination of safety review activities within the divisions; increase focus on medical error signal detection; increase epidemiological expertise to explore safety risks and signals in various population databases; and manage the increasing workload in ODS for new drug consultations and designing post-approval studies for new drug use in specific populations.

Finally, we plan to hire six FTEs to increase staff dedicated to evaluating and communicating drug safety risks to the health care community and the American public.

CONCLUSION

At FDA, providing the American public with safe and effective medical products is our core mission. We base decisions to approve a drug, or to keep it on the market if new safety findings surface, on a careful balancing of risk and benefit to patients. This is a multifaceted and complex decision process, involving scientific and public health issues. The recent initiatives we have announced will improve our current system to assess drug safety. Moreover, we will continue to evaluate new approaches to advance drug safety. As always, we value input from Congress, patients and the medical community as we develop and refine these drug safety initiatives.

While FDA can do its part by providing accurate information on drugs and working with drug manufacturers to withdraw drugs that cannot be used safely by physicians and their patients, ensuring the safest use of drugs that remain on the market is the greater challenge. Some adverse reactions are the result of medication errors related to circumstances outside of FDA jurisdiction, e.g., dispensing of drugs by pharmacists and prescribing by licensed health care providers regulated by the states. FDA recognizes that it has an important role to play in any larger process involving all interested parties, i.e., consumers, physicians, pharmacists, industry, and state regulators to address the challenge of ensuring the safest use of marketed drugs.

Once again, thank you for the opportunity to testify before the Committee today. I am happy to respond to questions.

Chairman TOM DAVIS. All right, thank you very much.

Let me start the questioning off. The label negotiation for Vioxx after the VIGOR study results took 6 months. What was going on for that period of time? What took the negotiations so long? In negotiations, both sides typically have to give up something to achieve a kind of resolution. Where was the FDA coming in, where was Merck coming in? What was going on here?

Dr. GALSON. The discussion that normally takes place between companies and a drug company, and in this case with Merck, what was going on was discussion about the specific label language that would go into the physician labeling for the drug. We were trying to work out exactly what was acceptable to both sides, putting pressure on Merck all the time to disclose the information that we thought most accurately represented——

Chairman TOM DAVIS. Can't you just dictate the disclosure?

Dr. GALSON. The label by law belongs to the product, which belongs to the company. So we can work together with them. We believe that most of the time we are very, very successful in getting what we want. One of the key facts about our new drug safety program is that we are going to make sure that information such as emerged in the VIGOR study is available to the public very, very quickly, even if the discussions with the company over the label are still taking place.

So we agree that these negotiations took longer than they should have. They took longer than is usual.

Chairman TOM DAVIS. What was the nature of the disagreement or the negotiations?

Dr. GALSON. It had to do with the specific language that was going to be used to describe the VIGOR study and the advice to health care practitioners.

Chairman TOM DAVIS. Have you produced any documents in terms of what was going on between you? Do we have that?

Dr. GALSON. Yes, we produced a lot of documents. We would be happy to point those out, including detailed descriptions.

Chairman TOM DAVIS. OK. Merck used a CV card as a promotional tool for Vioxx. Have you had a chance to review that card?

Dr. GALSON. I just saw it now.

Chairman TOM DAVIS. You've seen ours. It's tab five. I think you should have it in front of you under tab five. My question is going to be, is the information on the card accurate and what is your reaction to the information on the card?

Dr. GALSON. First of all, let me point out that our regulations on drug promotion have to do with making sure that the promotional materials are straightforward, are not false and misleading. We are able to require companies to put the same information in their promotional materials that are in the approved label.

In this particular case, since the label discussions were not completed, the company was not required to put the information on, except what was in their currently approved label. However, we think it is very important that the companies convey truthful information that is up to date with the scientific data that is available at the time.

Chairman Tom Davis. You don't see any illegality, then, in what they were putting out?

Dr. Galson. According to our regulations, no.

Chairman Tom Davis. OK.

Dr. Galson. We do think it is very important, and we are always willing to work with companies to talk about if they want to add information that is not in the label before it gets completed, we would do that.

Chairman Tom Davis. Would you say the information is accurate, or does this go along the lines of puffery, which often happens?

Dr. Galson. No, I think it was accurate based on the label, which is the legal standard that we use.

Dr. Galson. OK. How does the CDER plan to get the Office of Drug Safety more involved with the pre-approval of drugs and the post-surveillance of approved drugs?

Dr. Galson. Our new drug safety program creates a drug safety oversight board which includes equal membership from the Office of New Drugs and the Office of Drug Safety. What this board is going to do is look at emerging drug safety issues with particular drugs and decide when that information needs to be conveyed to the American public, even before it may reach the literature or before it gets in the label. So they will be sitting side by side with our Office of New Drugs in making these decisions and advising the Center as to when information needs to get posted on the Web site.

Chairman Tom Davis. Legalities aside, going back to the card, do you think it is accurate, what they were saying?

Dr. Galson. Well, it certainly did not reflect the information that was in the New England Journal, which is a very respected medical journal. So many physicians would say that it was not inclusive enough to really inform clinicians about the state of the literature.

Chairman Tom Davis. OK. I see my time is up. Mr. Waxman.

Mr. Waxman. Thank you, Mr. Chairman.

Dr. Galson, you just stated that the companies are permitted to use information on the label in their promotion. But the analyses in the cardiovascular card were not on the label. In fact, FDA objected to the presentation of data many times. Is that accurate?

Dr. Galson. I am sure we objected to the presentation of some data through the whole negotiation, yes. But I do not know about that particular data and how they were proposing that it be conveyed.

Again, our new program that we are proposing would have prevented this problem where the public and the practitioners were not aware of this information. So we think that we are addressing the sort of problem that happened here and making sure that it will not happen again.

Mr. Waxman. The card was based upon a pooled analysis of studies conducted prior to approval. Yet in discussing these studies, the FDA reviewer in 2001 stated that "The division has serious concerns with the combined analysis of different length and dosing regimens." What does that mean, different length and dosing regimens?

Dr. GALSON. It is very difficult when you are combining results from studies on humans, epidemiologic studies, to compare apples and oranges. So to really add data from different studies together, they have to be similar enough that it's scientifically valid to combine them. So that is what we were trying to convey, and it sounds like in that sentence.

Mr. WAXMAN. FDA also stated that "The data base overall includes short term low doses of Vioxx, only 265 patients have been taking Vioxx 50 milligrams for 6 months or more." Why was the FDA concerned about using a data base that consists of data from short term studies at low doses for safety assessment?

Dr. GALSON. Right. I think again, I was not one of the people sitting around the table having those discussions. But I can tell you what that was about was the idea that the effects of a drug, when given short term at low dose, are going to be different from the effects of a drug taken at high dose for a long period of time. So combining those types of studies is very problematic. That is, I am sure, what we were getting at.

Mr. WAXMAN. In contrast to the studies that were the basis of the cardiovascular card, the VIGOR study included 4,000 patients on Vioxx at 50 milligrams for approximately 9 months each. Which study is more informative on cardiovascular safety, the VIGOR study or the data base of pre-approval studies?

Dr. GALSON. I would say they are both valid. It depends whether the patient——

Mr. WAXMAN. Which is more informative?

Dr. GALSON. If you are taking the drug for a longer period of time, the longer study is more informative. If you are just taking a couple of doses after an injured tendon, a tendon injury, then the shorter one is OK.

Mr. WAXMAN. Let me hear from any of the gentlemen who have accompanied you, whether they have a thought on that. Which is more informative, a study of 4,000 patients on Vioxx at 50 milligrams for approximately 9 months, or this other study that included 265 patients taking Vioxx, 50 milligrams for 6 months or more?

Dr. JENKINS. Mr. Waxman, in general, longer studies are more informative.

Mr. WAXMAN. I am talking about the cardiovascular.

Dr. JENKINS. Yes. In general, longer studies at higher doses provide you additional information about the safety of a drug. But all studies have design features that you need to take into account. For example, the VIGOR study was an active control study. There was no placebo. So you are only comparing it to another drug. In the case of naproxen, we didn't really know exactly what the effects of naproxen would be.

The shorter term studies that you are referring to that were part of the NDA data base would have also included placebo. So they both provide useful information. Clearly a larger study, a longer term exposure gives you a lot more solid information about the drug.

Mr. WAXMAN. Could you turn to page 4? That page contains a graphic indicating that Vioxx may be 11 times safer than other anti-inflammatory medications. This graphic contains no assessment of statistical significance, no data on the actual numbers of deaths. It misstates the number of—I am talking about tab five. The graphic contains no assessment of statistical significance, no data on actual numbers of deaths, and it misstates the number of person years of analysis. It is based on a questionable pooled analysis of studies of varying lengths, doses and comparative drugs.

This week, my staff and the majority staff met with FDA to discuss these issues. At that meeting, an FDA drug reviewer told the staff that using this comparison with doctors is "scientifically inappropriate." Can you explain why Merck's use of the studies was scientifically inappropriate?

Dr. JENKINS. I'm sorry, did you ask me to explain why it was appropriate or inappropriate?

Mr. WAXMAN. Well, we were told by a representative from FDA that it was scientifically inappropriate. Why would he have reached that conclusion?

Dr. JENKINS. Well, obviously I can't speak for the reviewer that you spoke to earlier this week. But I think some of the concerns that would be raised include combining studies of different durations, different doses, different patient populations. One factor here is they have combined, apparently, numerous non-steroidal agents rather than showing the individual agents that might have been studied. This is not the type of presentation of the data that we would include in the labeling. And what you have told me, we did not include this presentation in the labeling.

Mr. WAXMAN. So the presentation is information that was not on the label.

Let me just ask one last question, if I might, Mr. Chairman. You have been criticized about the information that was provided to FDA prior to dissemination. Although FDA receives tens of thousands of pages of promotional materials from drug companies and only does spot checks on them, we learned yesterday FDA does not know whether it reviewed the accuracy of the cardiovascular card. I assume that is probably an accurate statement, given all the promotional data you have to review and the few resources you have to do it, which I think highlights a point that we ought to take into consideration if we expect FDA to do their job.

Thank you, Mr. Chairman.

Chairman TOM DAVIS. Thank you.

Mr. Gutknecht.

Mr. GUTKNECHT. Thank you, Mr. Chairman, for having this hearing. I thank the gentlemen for coming to testify.

Let me just say first, though, I think there are two central questions in this debate, and I think it is an ongoing debate about the role the FDA plays and the responsibilities that they have and the drug companies have. The first question is, just who is the FDA protecting? Second question is, what are the ethical responsibilities of companies like Merck?

It seems to me, based on just what we have learned so far this morning, that both the FDA and the pharmaceutical companies sort of miss the mark. Even the response, with all due respect, to the question about the card and operation victory, or, I'm sorry, it's Project Offense, it strikes me that there is a disconnect here. Because on one hand you say, well, that card is technically legal. But is that ethical? Isn't there a role for ethics to play here?

In other words, if you look at the Enron scandal, and a lot of scandals the United States has been through over the last several years, essentially they all come down to, well, the law didn't say we had to and therefore we didn't have to. Isn't that correct?

Dr. GALSON. I do not want to comment on the other scandals. But I can tell you that of course, ethics is a very, very important part of all the work that we do at FDA. But as you know, as a regulatory agency, we have to follow the letter of the law and our regulations. There are limits on the powers of the FDA. We do think that the steps that we are taking that were announced by Secretary Leavitt in February are going to go a long way toward addressing a lot of concerns about communication and about early information, and as well with the promotion issue.

Mr. GUTKNECHT. Well, let me just ask about this, because you are probably familiar with the article that appeared in the New York Times February 25th in which they claim, and apparently it is correct, that at least 10 of the 32 Government drug advisors who last week endorsed continued marketing of the huge selling painkillers Celebrex, Bextra and Vioxx had consulted with the drug industries over the last few years. They go on to say that if the 10 advisors had not cast their votes, the committee would have voted 12 to 8 that Bextra should be withdrawn and 14 to 8 that Vioxx should not return to the market. Are you familiar with that article, and does that cause any concern at the FDA?

Dr. GALSON. Yes, I am familiar with the article. The issue of financial conflict of interest with our advisory committee members, which is really what you are getting at, is a very, very complex issue. The way that we do conflict of interest screening and selection of our members is governed by the Trade Secrets Act, the Federal advisory committee rules, the Freedom of Information Act. We follow, as do all the Federal agencies, the same rules in screening people.

We do not agree with the assessment that the members of the committee were so conflicted that they could not give us neutral advice. What we have found throughout the years is that we need, and the public expects us to have the very, very best people on our advisory committee. Because of the prevalence of doing pharmaceutical research in our medical schools, it is very, very difficult for us to find the experts that we need and that you all deserve on our committees who have never done any work.

So the judgment about how we screen those people and when we decide to have a conflict and when we feel that we can waive them is the subject of many regulations, as I mentioned. We do think this is an important issue, though, so we are continuing to look at this question. We are actively looking at how we do the financial conflicts and the conflicts of interest and we will continue to work with you and discuss it with you more.

Mr. GUTKNECHT. Mr. Chairman, I would at least like to submit this for the record. I would ask unanimous consent that it go into the record.

Chairman TOM DAVIS. Without objection, that will go into the record.

[The information referred to follows:]

10 Voters on Panel Backing Pain Pills Had Industry Ties

By GARDINER HARRIS and ALEX BERENSON

Ten of the 32 government drug advisers who last week endorsed continued marketing of the huge-selling pain pills Celebrex, Bextra and Vioxx have consulted in recent years for the drugs' makers, according to disclosures in medical journals and other public records.

If the 10 advisers had not cast their votes, the committee would have voted 12 to 8 that Bextra should be withdrawn and 14 to 8 that Vioxx should not return to the market. The 10 advisers with company ties voted 9 to 1 to keep Bextra on the market and 9 to 1 for Vioxx's return.

The votes of the 10 did not substantially influence the committee's decision on Celebrex because only one committee member voted that Celebrex should be withdrawn.

Eight of the 10 members said in interviews that their past relationships with the drug companies had not influenced their votes. The two others did not respond to phone or e-mail messages.

Researchers with ties to industry commonly serve on Food and Drug Administration advisory panels, but their presence has long been a contentious issue.

The agency has said it tries to balance expertise - often found among those who have conducted clinical trials of the drugs in question or otherwise studied them - with potential conflicts of interest.

Several of the panel members flagged with conflicts said most or all of the money went not to themselves but to their universities or institutions.

The Center for Science in the Public Interest, an advocacy group in Washington that maintains a large database of scientists' industry ties culled from disclosures in medical journals and other public documents, analyzed the panel members' affiliations at the request of The New York Times.

The center has been a frequent critic of the F.D.A. and of the pharmaceutical industry. The center's analysis may understate the industry ties of the panel participants because some ties may not have been previously disclosed publicly.

Dr. Sheldon Krimsky, a science policy expert at Tufts University, said such conflicts were common on F.D.A. advisory panels. The agency often conceals these conflicts, and studies have shown that, taken as a whole, money does influence scientific judgments, Dr. Krimsky said.

He added, "F.D.A. has to work harder to fill panels with people without conflicts, and if they feel they have the best committee, they at least ought to make it transparent."

But Dan Troy, a Washington lawyer who was until last year the agency's general counsel, said that finding knowledgeable experts without financial conflicts was difficult. Suggesting that such conflicts skew a panel's decisions "buys into an overly conspiratorial view of the world," Mr. Troy said.

A spokeswoman for the F.D.A. said no one at the agency would comment on specific panel members' industry ties.

Before each of three meetings of the advisory board last week, an agency secretary read a statement absolving panel members of conflicts of interest because the committee's agenda involved "issues of broad applicability and there are no products being approved."

The secretary also said, "The Food and Drug Administration acknowledges that there may be potential conflicts of interest, but because of the general nature of the discussions before the committee, these potential conflicts are mitigated."

But the committee took nine votes, three for each drug, on whether Celebrex, Bextra or Vioxx hurt the heart, should continue to be marketed and, if so, under what restrictions. These votes were deeply important to the three companies - Merck, Pfizer and Novartis - that came before the committee. Indeed, shares of Merck and Pfizer soared last Friday after the panel's votes.

Ten members of the panel have worked in some capacity in recent years for Merck, the maker of Vioxx; Pfizer, the maker of Celebrex and Bextra; or Novartis, which is applying to sell Prexige, a very similar pill discussed by the panel, according to the public disclosures.

An 11th panel member, Dr. Jack Cush, a rheumatologist at Presbyterian Hospital in Dallas, said a disclosure that he once consulted for Pfizer was incorrect, so he was excluded from the analysis.

Of the 30 votes cast by the 10 panel members on whether Celebrex, Bextra and Vioxx should continue to be marketed, 28 favored the drugs. Among the 66 votes cast by the remaining 22 members of the panel, just 37 favored the drugs.

Dr. Steven Abramson, a rheumatologist at New York University School of Medicine who was on the panel, has consulted for Pfizer and Novartis. "The F.D.A. is looking for people who understand the science behind these medicines," and such an understanding often results from working with drug makers, he said.

Dr. John Farrar, a neurologist at the University of Pennsylvania who has received research support from Pfizer and is a panel member, agreed. "I think F.D.A. would have a hard time finding people who are good at what they do who never spoke to a pharmaceutical company," he said.

But Dr. Curt Furberg, a panel member and an epidemiologist at Wake Forest University who had no ties to any of the drug companies, said he was "uncomfortable with the Pfizer-friendly undertone" at the meeting. And he worried that Pfizer's financial relationships with some panel members might have played a role in setting that tone.

Joan Wainwright, a spokeswoman for Merck, said the company had had no role in choosing any of the scientists on the panel.

Merck has made no decision on whether it will reintroduce Vioxx, Ms. Wainwright said. "We look forward to discussing the outcomes of the meeting with the F.D.A. and other regulatory authorities," she said.

Andy McCormick, a spokesman for Pfizer, said the company had no plans to withdraw Bextra from the market. He also said that Pfizer had played no role in helping to choose the panel.

Critics of the drug industry said they were not surprised that the panel's decisions would have been different if scientists with financial ties to the companies had recused themselves from the votes.

"My employees usually vote for me as well," said W. Mark Lanier, a lawyer in Houston who represents people who have sued Merck after taking Vioxx and suffering heart attacks or strokes.

Some lawyers and Wall Street analysts said last week that the panel's decision would help to protect Merck and Pfizer from lawsuits. But juries will be more skeptical of the decision after they learn about the composition of the panel, Mr. Lanier said.

Christopher A. Seeger, a lawyer in New York with many Vioxx clients, said the fact that scientists had not recused themselves simply highlighted the close ties between the drug industry and academic researchers. He said researchers were afraid to say anything negative about new drugs because doing so might jeopardize their chances of participating in clinical trials and publishing papers.

Several panel members said the important split on the committee was not so much between those with industry ties and those who did not have those ties but between experts who treat arthritis patients and those who do not.

Dr. Cush was angry that the voices of the panel's rheumatologists were nearly drowned out by statisticians and others who do not have to cope with anguished patients every day.

Dr. Furberg said clinicians often wanted access to therapies without understanding the devastating public health consequences of their prescribing decisions. Celebrex, Bextra and Vioxx have never been proved in clinical trials to cure pain any better than ibuprofen or more than a dozen other, older pain pills.

"Fifty patients a day probably die from those drugs, and who is speaking for them?" Dr. Furberg said.

Dr. Alastair Wood, an associate dean at Vanderbilt University and the panel's chairman, said he was disappointed that the F.D.A. failed to disclose the financial conflicts of the panel's participants before each day's meeting.

"I'm a great believer in letting it all hang out," he said.

Still, Dr. Wood said that even with its conflicts the panel was a tough critic of the drugs. Many of the panel members who were among the narrow majorities approving continued marketing of Bextra and Vioxx did so only with the stipulation that severe restrictions be imposed on their uses, he noted.

He said he expected that the uses of the drugs would be confined to very limited patient populations.

Mr. GUTKNECHT. Let me just give you another example of how the FDA does not always act in a timely—I would like to submit for the record a letter that I sent to the FDA 8 months ago, asking for information about the facilities that are FDA approved around the country; 8 months ago. Just last Friday, maybe because we are having this hearing today, I finally got an answer. That is just one example. It amazes me that it takes the FDA so long to get to the heart of this, and more importantly, that there is this sort of ongoing ethical dilemma of how we are going to deal with these things.

Let me give you another example. The FDA spends an awful lot of time and effort determining whether or not Americans ought to be able to buy drugs from other countries. Can you tell me which of these two packages came from Canada and which came from the United States?

[The information referred to follows:]

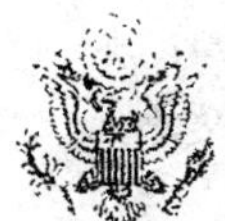

GIL GUTKNECHT
1st District, Minnesota

gil@mail.house.gov
www.gil.house.gov

COMMITTEE ASSIGNMENTS

AGRICULTURE

Chairman, Subcommittee on
Department Operations, Oversight,
Nutrition and Forestry

SCIENCE
Vice Chairman

BUDGET

Congress of the United States
House of Representatives
Washington, DC 20515–2301

August 17, 2004

Jeremiah Kelly
Congressional Affairs Specialist
Food and Drug Administration
5600 Fishers Lane
Rockville MD 20857-0001

Dear Mr. Kelly,

I am writing today to request information related to FDA-approved pharmaceutical manufacturing facilities outside of the United States.

I would like a list of all such facilities, including that city and country in which they are located and the date on which they were last inspected. The most recent information on this that my staff has been able to find is located in a CBO report dated March, 1998, with information on inspections in 1996.

I thank you for your attention to this matter and look forward to your reply.

Sincerely,

Gil Gutknecht
Member of Congress

HOME OFFICE
Midway Office Plaza
1530 Greenview Drive SW, Suite #108
Rochester, MN 55902
(507) 252-9841
(507) 252-9915 Fax

109 East Second Street
Fairmont, MN 56031
(507) 238-2835
(507) 238-1405 Fax

425 Cannon House Office Building
Washington, DC 20515-2301
(202) 225-2472
(202) 225-3246 Fax

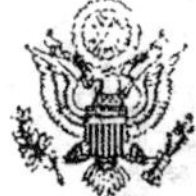

GIL GUTKNECHT
1ST DISTRICT, MINNESOTA

Congress of the United States
House of Representatives
Washington, DC 20515–2301

December 9, 2004

Lester Crawford
Acting Commissioner
Food and Drug Administration
5600 Fishers Lane
Rockville MD 20857-0001

Dear Commissioner Crawford,

I am writing today to follow up on a request that was faxed to the Office of Congressional Affairs on August 17, 2004. As of the date of this correspondence, I have not received a response to my request.

My staff initially inquired with the Office of Congressional Affairs regarding a list our office was seeking. In fact, we were directed to send the correspondence via fax and hard copy to a specific specialist in your agency. Three months later, we have not received a response. In fact, my staff has followed up with Mr. Jeremiah Kelly and Ms. Liz Ortuzar on several occasions for a status update where, frankly, we have been given a multitude of excuses why a response has not been provided. Moreover, my office has contacted various personnel time and time again, but we have not received a response. I am very unsatisfied with the fashion in which my office has been dealt with in connection with this matter. I hope you do not believe that Members of Congress should wait more than three months for a response.

For your convenience, I have attached the original correspondence for your review. My request was for a list of FDA-inspected pharmaceutical manufacturing facilities outside of the United States, including the city and country in which each is located and the date on which they each last inspected. I would also like to know what product is manufactured in each facility and who owns each facility. This seems like information your office would be able to get rather quickly due to the nature of request.

I thank you for your attention to this matter and look forward to your reply.

Sincerely,

Gil Gutknecht
Member of Congress

WASHINGTON OFFICE
425 CANNON HOUSE OFFICE BUILDING
WASHINGTON, DC 20515-2301
(202) 225-2472
(202) 225-3246 FAX
gil@mail.house.gov
www.gil.house.gov

PRINTED ON RECYCLED PAPER

HOME OFFICE
MIDWAY OFFICE PLAZA
1530 GREENVIEW DRIVE SW, SUITE #108
ROCHESTER, MN 55902
(507) 252-9841
(507) 252-9915 FAX
IN MN: 1-800-862-8632 TOLL FREE

Dr. GALSON. No, sir.

Mr. GUTKNECHT. Well, in truth of the matter, neither one of them. They were both from the United States. I will be honest about that. But the important thing is, these were free samples that were given to people here in the United States after both the drug companies and the FDA knew that there were serious potential health problems with these drugs and the FDA and the drug company was doing nothing to inform the consumers.

There is no warning on these. Consumers were taking these drugs long after you knew and the company knew that there were potential health risks.

So it really does come back to that basic question. You started your remarks today by saying the FDA is the gold standard for the world. OK. It strikes me then that we have a moral and ethical responsibility to make certain that physicians and consumers are warned about the safety of these drugs. When you withhold information, particularly from physicians about that, it seems to me that it does begin to weaken that gold standard, doesn't it?

Dr. GALSON. We are not in the business of withholding information. We have to follow our regulations in terms of protecting trade secrets and commercial confidential information. We are working with our new initiatives to do better at getting information out early to consumers when it is needed.

On the importation issue, I think you know we have been working closely with Congress and we continue to do that. We do have some safety concerns about imported medicines. But you said those are not imported.

Chairman TOM DAVIS. The gentleman's time has expired. I thank you very much.

The gentleman from Maryland.

Mr. CUMMINGS. Thank you very much, Mr. Chairman.

I am simply fascinated by all of this. I must say that as a former user of Vioxx, I am very, very concerned. But I am even more concerned about my constituents. We have one of the highest, in the Seventh Congressional District of Maryland, one of the highest heart attack and sudden death from heart attack rates in the country. We have a lot of people who I'm sure have used Vioxx.

So I say all that to ask these questions. Dr. Jenkins, let me ask you this. There have been numerous questions about the cardiovascular card, so you are familiar with it, are you not?

Dr. JENKINS. I have seen it today, yes.

Mr. CUMMINGS. Is this the first time you saw it?

Dr. JENKINS. Yes.

Mr. CUMMINGS. So you know what it says, then?

Dr. JENKINS. I received a copy of it this morning, so I reviewed it this morning.

Mr. CUMMINGS. What are these cards used for, sir?

Dr. JENKINS. I can't say for sure how this card was used. But I'm assuming, based on the front page, which says, in response to your questions, that this would be provided to physicians to give them information about Vioxx.

Mr. CUMMINGS. Now, you're familiar with the VIGOR study, are you not?

Dr. JENKINS. Yes.

Mr. CUMMINGS. And when you look at what is on this card, is it consistent with the VIGOR study?

Dr. JENKINS. This card, as I read it, does not present any information related to the VIGOR study. This card is presenting information from trials in osteoarthritis patients that were conducted before approval of the drug. The VIGOR study, to my read, is not mentioned in this card.

Mr. CUMMINGS. Now, would you feel comfortable giving this card to a doctor, let's say prior to the time that Vioxx was taken off the market?

Dr. JENKINS. Well, I think as Dr. Galson said, we feel that it is important for the companies to provide fair and balanced information. So the information that is in this card does not present the entire picture about Vioxx at that time. I don't know exactly when this card was in use. But if it was in use after the VIGOR study, we think it would be very important to alert doctors to the data from that study. I would note that study was publicly available starting in March 2000. So it was not as if physicians had not been made aware of the data.

Mr. CUMMINGS. So if the doctors in my district were presented with this study by Merck, and said, this is Vioxx, it is something that is good for your patients, that they have a less likely chance of developing some cardiovascular problems based upon this study if they prescribe Vioxx for their patients, that statement would be inaccurate, is that right, or accurate? What would you say?

Dr. JENKINS. Well, I don't know how this card was presented. They presented the data. I don't know if they said, you know, it is elevenfold less likely to cause death. The data are in the table. I don't know how the card was used. I don't know how it was presented. I think it would be important for doctors not to rely solely on the information in this card in making their prescribing decisions for patients.

Mr. CUMMINGS. Let's go back to my colleague on the other side who just asked some questions. One of the things that we are most concerned about is the integrity of the system. That is, when we are, if taxpayers are spending their tax dollars to see that an organization like the FDA is providing them with information that is accurate, and we want to know, as Members of this Congress, that the information that our constituents and their doctors are getting is accurate, is that a reasonable expectation, do you think?

Dr. GALSON. Absolutely.

Mr. CUMMINGS. I can't hear you.

Dr. GALSON. Absolutely, yes.

Mr. CUMMINGS. So at what point do you all come in, I mean, if you find out that inaccurate information is being presented to doctors, and information that could lead, literally, to fatalities, I mean, you talked about all these things that you now have in place, how do we make sure that didn't happen back then, and now how do we make sure that it does not happen in the future based upon what you are about, the plans that you just talked about?

The things that I am most concerned about is that I don't want people in my district or anywhere in this world taking drugs that can lead them to heart attacks, and then they're getting inaccurate information. That's crazy. And we are paying for it.

Chairman TOM DAVIS. The gentleman's time has expired.

Mr. Marchant, the gentleman from Texas.

Mr. MARCHANT. I have a question. Can the clinical studies conducted to support approval of the drug product identify every risk associated with that product when it is approved and becomes widely available? How does the FDA manage this lack of definitive risk data?

Dr. GALSON. That is a really excellent point. We can't predict all side effects from drugs based on the studies that we get before a drug is approved. Because the studies are not large enough to detect all of the problems that may take place once the drug goes into larger population, for one.

Two, the population that takes place, that participates in the clinical trials is not the same as the general U.S. population. So drugs are going to be used by different people. Third, a drug may not be used according to the instructions on the label, so the side effects may be different.

Mr. MARCHANT. What are the effects of a drug that is designed and made for one purpose but doctors discover other purposes for that drug and begin to prescribe those drugs, not for the purpose by which they were tested, but for purposes that they have discovered they can achieve with some other illness? And how do they affect your testing down the road and is that ever a factor in your testing?

Dr. GALSON. Yes. This happens all the time. It is a natural part of a drug's cycle. What a pharmaceutical company can do is come back to us after a drug is approved for one purpose and ask that it be approved for another purpose if they have studies that demonstrate that the drug is effective in that second purpose. So the label can be modified to include new uses down the line.

Sometimes drugs are used by individual physicians for what we call off-label uses as well, even when they are not approved, though.

Mr. MARCHANT. Do you have situations where the original use of the drug turns out to be quite effective and does not have any long-term negative benefits, but then the secondary use that's brought in then runs into trouble? Does that tank the entire drug, then, when the secondary use comes in and is exposed?

Dr. GALSON. Right. That particular example has certainly happened, and there are lots of variances as well. There have been drugs that we have changed the labeling on because of this use that's not according to the label to make sure that people are aware if there are drug safety issues that have arisen that they may occur with this use that is not on the label.

With our new program, we feel that we will be better able to inform the public about these off-label side effects when they do occur.

Mr. MARCHANT. Do you have the powers, the police powers or administrative powers to make sure that the thousands of boxes of samples that are sitting on doctors' shelves are either turned back in or not continued to be given out?

Dr. GALSON. Yes.

Mr. MARCHANT. What kind of a period can you make a decision 1 day and have doctors informed enough to quit using that product?

Mr. MARCHANT. The samples that physicians use in their office are subject to regulations from the FDA. Of course, they are not allowed to give out expired medication. There is a date stamped on all those samples. They would have to stop giving them out at that point.

Mr. MARCHANT. Is there a step beyond that where the doctor has an obligation to contact the patient, or do you just let those prescriptions expire?

Dr. GALSON. The regulations cover the point at which the drug is given out. So if someone has it in their medicine cabinet and it expires, it is up to us as patients to make sure that it is not past the expiration point.

Mr. MARCHANT. OK, thank you very much.

Chairman TOM DAVIS. Thank you very much.

Mr. Towns.

Mr. TOWNS. Thank you very much, Mr. Chairman.

Let me begin with you, Dr. Jenkins. Does FDA have the authority to require a manufacturer to conduct clinical trials after approval?

Dr. JENKINS. In certain situations, we do have that authority. For example, under the Best Pharmaceuticals for Children Act that was passed a couple of years ago, we have the authority to require studies in children for approved drugs. In other cases, the authority is a little less clear. But we feel like we have the ability to strongly encourage and work with companies to get them to do the studies that we think need to be done after approval.

There are also situations where we can require studies be done after approval under parts of our regulations, such as when we approve a product under what we call accelerated approval, there is a requirement that the companies followup with a confirmatory clinical trial after approval. So there are situations when we have the regulatory authority to require companies to do studies. There are other situations where our ability to require studies is not so clear, but we clearly work with companies to encourage them to do those studies.

Mr. TOWNS. How would the negotiation take place? Can you just walk me through that?

Dr. JENKINS. I'm sorry, I could not hear you.

Mr. TOWNS. How would the negotiation take place? How would you bring about this?

Dr. JENKINS. To get them to do a study?

Mr. TOWNS. Yes.

Dr. JENKINS. There are several scenarios. But I am assuming you are talking about in the post-approval period, if we became aware of a new situation in the post-approval period that we felt warranted additional study, we would meet with the company and advise them of what we thought needed to be done. We might try to get them to agree to what we call a post-marketing study commitment, which is a written commitment from the company to do a study that actually has a time line from when they will initiate the study and when they will complete it. We would review any protocol that they would submit for that study and give them feedback about the adequacy of the study and how it was going to be conducted.

Mr. TOWNS. Thank you.

Does the agency currently require that ads for new drug products receive pre-market approval?

Dr. GALSON. No.

Mr. TOWNS. If this entire class of Cox–2 drugs were banned from the market, aren't steroids and narcotics one of the few treatment options that do not result in gastrointestinal problems which would be available to patients with chronic pain?

Dr. GALSON. When we made our announcement about changes in the regulatory status of this class of drugs, it was with the recognition that patients with pain need a wide variety of medications because of the different circumstances that each patient has, both their medical condition, their pre-existing conditions, other drugs that they are taking. So we really think it is important that a wide variety of medication classes are available. There is not enough out there for pain. There is a clear recognition of that.

Mr. TOWNS. Isn't one of the principal reasons that the advisory council supported continuing the availability of Cox–2 drugs the fact that they present a reduced risk for GI problems in patients?

Dr. GALSON. That was definitely one of the considerations that the advisory committee looked at, and one of the things that we looked at as well.

Mr. TOWNS. Some have argued that alternative therapies are available to Vioxx users. Merck even believed that this was true when they withdrew the product. Given patient reaction, would it not be fair to say that there are many patients with chronic pain who have been unable to find any comparable substitute medication?

Dr. GALSON. We do not have any formal way of answering that question. Anecdotally, though, we have heard complaints from patients who felt that they had tried other medications and that either Vioxx or Bextra was the only thing that worked. We think that the current availability of the one drug that is left in that class in the United States, Celebrex, is addressing most of this problem.

But there is a lot of variability between different people in which drugs work. We think we have a lot of research that is taking place, funded by the Government and the industry, to look at why certain people react better to one drug or another drug. Hopefully in the future, we will be better able to target which drugs work best with certain patients.

Chairman TOM DAVIS. The gentleman's time has expired.

Mr. TOWNS. Thank you, Mr. Chairman.

[The prepared statement of Hon. Edolphus Towns follows:]

OPENING STATEMENT
BY
HON. ED TOWNS (D-NY)
FOR
FULL GOVERNMENT REFORM COMMITTEE HEARING ON
"Risk and Responsibility: The Roles of FDA and Pharmaceutical Companies in
Ensuring the Safety of Approved Drugs, Like Vioxx"

MAY 5, 2005

MR. CHAIRMAN, TODAY'S HEARING RAISES IMPORTANT ISSUES ABOUT HOW THE FOOD AND DRUG ADMINISTRATION SHOULD APPROACH ISSUES OF DRUG SAFETY.

THE TEST CASE WE ARE CONSIDERING CONCERNS VIOXX, A PAIN MEDICATION PREVIOUSLY PRESCRIBED FOR ARTHRITIS PATIENTS AND OTHERS WHO SUFFER FROM CHRONIC PAIN. THIS MEDICATION IS ONE THAT MANY PATIENTS AND PHYSICIANS WOULD ARGUE HAS NO EFFECTIVE SUBSTITUTE. AND IN FACT, IT IS THE ONLY DRUG THERAPY THAT HAS BEEN APPROVED FOR JUVENILE RHEUMATOID ARTHRITIS WHICH AFFLICTS SOME 300,000 CHILDREN. SO WHILE ARTHRITIS IS RARELY THOUGHT OF AS A LIFE-THREATENING ILLNESS, I THINK IT IS IMPORTANT TO SHARE SOME FACTS ABOUT JUST HOW DEVASTATING THIS DISEASE REALLY IS.

--43 MILLION AMERICANS HAVE BEEN DIAGNOSED WITH ARTHRITIS;
--23 MILLION HAVE POSSIBLE CHRONIC JOINT SYMPTOMS;
--AMERICANS WITH RHEUMATOID ARTHRITIS FACE A SIGNIFICANTLY INCREASED RATE OF CARDIOVASCULAR DISEASE; AND
--IN FACT, 9,500 AMERICANS DID DIE FROM ARTHRITIS IN 2003.

MANY HAVE ARGUED THAT ALTERNATIVES TO VIOXX DO EXIST. YET WE FIND THAT MANY OF THESE TRADITIONAL OVER-THE-COUNTER PAIN KILLERS COULD LEAD TO SERIOUS STOMACH

PROBLEMS, LIKE BLEEDING ULCERS. THESE AILMENTS CAUSE OVER 100,000 HOSPITALIZATIONS ANNUALLY AND REPORTEDLY 16,000 DEATHS.

GIVEN THESE FACTS, ONE MUST ASK THE QUESTION IS CHRONIC PAIN, WHICH CAN LEAD TO IMMOBILITY, BETTER THAN THE RISK OF HEART PROBLEMS? MANY PHYSICIANS HAVE COME DOWN ON THE SIDE OF MAINTAINING THEIR PATIENTS' MOBILITY. AND MANY PATIENTS, IN TESTIMONY TO THE F.D.A., STRESSED THAT VIOXX RESTORED THEIR QUALITY OF LIFE.

ONE THING IS CERTAINLY CLEAR: FDA NEEDS MORE AUTHORITY TO ADDRESS PROBLEMS THAT ARISE AFTER DRUGS REACH THE MARKET. HOPEFULLY, TODAY'S HEARING WILL ASSIST US AND THE AGENCY IN DETERMINING HOW BEST TO REQUIRE LABEL CHANGES AND ADDITIONAL RESEARCH FROM COMPANIES. CERTAINLY, WE NEED TO ACTIVELY CONSIDER NEW AUTHORITY IN THIS AREA FOR THE OFFICE OF NEW DRUGS. WE ALSO NEED TO BE MINDFUL OF THE BENEFITS AS WELL AS THE RISKS FOR THERAPIES THAT IMPROVE THE QUALITY OF LIFE FOR PATIENTS WITH CHRONIC CONDITIONS. LIKEWISE WE NEED TO REMEMBER THAT NO DRUG IS RISK-FREE AND THERE WILL BE SOME PATIENTS WHO ARE NOT ABLE TO TAKE CERTAIN MEDICATIONS BECAUSE OF THE PARTICULAR NEGATIVE SIDE EFFECTS ON THEM, SIDE EFFECTS, WHICH MAY NOT AFFECT ALL PATIENTS.

MR. CHAIRMAN, I LOOK FORWARD TO HEARING FROM THE WITNESSES TODAY ON THIS VERY IMPORTANT HEALTH ISSUE WHICH CAN HOPEFULLY HELP US TO COME TO A RESPONSIBLE APPROACH IN OUR EFFORTS TO IMPROVE DRUG SAFETY.

Chairman TOM DAVIS. Thank you very much.

Mrs. Foxx.

Mrs. FOXX. Thank you, Mr. Chairman.

Would you tell us what has been the most valuable lesson you have learned from this process and what changes are going to accrue from those lessons?

Dr. GALSON. Sure. The most important lesson that we have taken from what has happened with the anti-inflammatory drugs and as well with the antidepressant drugs that you have heard so much about is that the American public, both practitioners and patients, want to get clear, accurate information as early as possible. They want this information so that they can participate in their own health care decisions. Physicians want it so they can provide high quality advice to their patients.

We feel like the steps that Commissioner Crawford and Secretary Leavitt have taken to set up the Drug Safety Board, to bring people from across the FDA and people from outside the agency in to help us make these decisions on when to put the information out into the public and then to set up a mechanism to do that on our Web site and with specific, succinct information products is really going to make a big difference and go a long way toward addressing the lessons of the last year with these drugs.

Chairman TOM DAVIS. Any other questions?

Mr. WAXMAN. Would the gentlelady yield?

Chairman TOM DAVIS. Would you yield to Mr. Waxman?

Mrs. FOXX. Sure.

Chairman TOM DAVIS. She had an additional minute and a half.

Mr. WAXMAN. OK. It is a question I wanted to ask Dr. Jenkins, and I appreciate the opportunity to do it.

Dr. Jenkins, you said that there ought to be a complete presentation to a doctor. One year after the VIGOR study, Merck representatives were told to state, "Doctor, as you can see, cardiovascular mortality is reported in over 6,000 patients was Vioxx 0.1 versus NSAIDs 0.8 versus placebo 0." This is 1 year after the VIGOR study. In other words, they're saying that even though their own VIGOR study showed that Vioxx was five times more dangerous, they are making a representation that Vioxx is eight times safer.

Do you think that was a fair and complete and balanced presentation for a representative to give to a doctor?

Dr. JENKINS. As I said earlier, I believe that you do need to provide balanced presentation. It would be important to include information about the VIGOR trial once that became available. It was publicly announced, I believe, in March 2000. It was published in the New England Journal.

So physicians could have been aware or should have been aware of that data. But I don't know that I can support the idea of not making it part of the company's presentation to physicians. Whether they are legally required to do that, I think Dr. Galson addressed that earlier. But I think it is important that they provide balanced information.

Mr. WAXMAN. And that is not balanced information, that presentation?

Dr. JENKINS. I think it would be important to include the information about the VIGOR trial.

Mr. WAXMAN. Thank you.

Chairman TOM DAVIS. I thank the gentleman.

The gentlelady from California.

Ms. WATSON. Thank you so much, Mr. Chairman.

I was going to yield some time—OK, thank you very much.

The subject of this hearing today, and I thank the Chair for bringing it into focus, is the role of FDA and pharmaceutical companies in ensuring the safety of approved drugs. Then they give you one, like Vioxx. Well, I have another concern and this I will direct toward Dr. Galson.

My concern, and I do have legislation in regarding dental amalgam fillings, is that these fillings are comprised of over 50 percent mercury, the most toxic substance known. And it is impacted in a filling that goes into the mouth of children and pregnant women, and we know the harm that can be done.

For ages, we have been asking the FDA to look into the use of mercury in the amalgam. And we have not had definitive, empirical evidence as to the harm mercury amalgams can do in the human body. Can you shed some light why for over the last 20 years there has been a failure to classify mercury-containing amalgam fillings as harmful?

Dr. GALSON. Ma'am, the part of the agency that I am responsible for is the drug part. The amalgam fillings are regulated by the Center for Devices, which I am not responsible for. But I will make sure that you get information responsive to your question and set up meetings, if that is needed.

Ms. WATSON. I would very much appreciate that. If you could direct a letter to me as to what your action plan is, and then direct the question to whatever agency is responsible, I would appreciate it.

Dr. GALSON. Absolutely.

Ms. WATSON. Thank you very much, Mr. Chairman.

Mr. WAXMAN. Would the gentlelady yield, since she has more time?

Ms. WATSON. Yes.

[The prepared statement of Hon. Diane E. Watson follows:]

Statement by Congresswoman Diane E. Watson
Government Reform Hearing: Risk and Responsibility –
Roles of FDA and Pharmaceutical Companies in Ensuring
the Safety of Approved Drugs, like Vioxx
May 5, 2005

Thank you Mr. Chairman.

I would like to raise another point that must be considered by the next Commissioner of the FDA. It is a situation that is as serious as the Vioxx question and even more widespread than a niche drug. I am speaking about dental Amalgam filling that is comprised of over 50% mercury. Mercury is a known neuro-toxic substance. The effects of mercury are harmful, especially in pregnant women and small children. The fact that fillings are placed in every age group of the country provides justified apprehension. The FDA has refused to classify this mercury containing dental device and continues to sidestep the issue today.

Mr. Chairman I am concerned with the negative implications evident in the drug approval process when industry money, conflict of interest, or bias is present. One way to study the safety of marketed drugs and widely used devices is through transparent studies conducted in large clinical databases.

Regarding amalgam, a concern that raises a red flag, whenever the FDA is questioned they point to a large study that they have commissioned to study the effects of Amalgam. The studies they refer to are subject to some of the same problems in the approval process that I have mentioned above. The FDA is looking to hang their hats on a study from a orphanage in Portugal, which was investigated in the past 2 years for indiscretions with the children, and a study in a low income areas of Boston and Maine, in which the subjects families are compensated for the placement of mercury containing amalgam in their mouths, and the disclosure is vague if at all.

Mr. Chairman I commend this Government Reform investigation in to drug safety and I support the effort to recommend amendments to current FDA procedure. Further, I hope that the Committee will investigate the over 20 year failure of the FDA to classify mercury containing Amalgam fillings. Additionally, we should request the Agency to show the American public why the last known use of mercury in the human body is safe.

Mr. WAXMAN. I want to go back to that give and take of the FDA negotiating changes in the label with the company. It seems like you had what you thought ought to be disclosed and the company did not quite agree with it, and you are not in a position legally to order it, even though you thought the public and the doctors ought to have this, particularly the doctors ought to have this warning information in light of the new studies.

Dr. GALSON. Right.

Mr. WAXMAN. Do you recall what you had to give up that the company wanted you to give up?

Dr. GALSON. I was not one of the participants around the table in this discussion. So that is kind of first-hand knowledge that somebody who was sitting there would have to have.

Mr. WAXMAN. Well, some of the documents pointed it out, and maybe Dr. Jenkins can answer this. But the Kaplan-Meyer curve, maybe you can tell us about it, that was not included. And the label perhaps most important to Merck, the label included the statement that "the significance of the cardiovascular findings of these three studies, VIGOR and two placebo-controlled studies, is unknown." Now, that was something the FDA did not want but the company did, is that right?

Dr. JENKINS. Mr. Waxman, I was also not directly involved with the discussions between the agency and Merck about the labeling for the VIGOR trial. I have read some of the documents that you are referring to, and I think there were complex issues about how the data was to be analyzed and how the data was to be presented in the labeling.

I know there were differences of opinion between the agency reviewers and the sponsor regarding, for example, whether the risk changed over time, meaning the longer you were on the drug, did the risk go up or down, based on the results from the trial. That was part of the discussion about whether the data should be presented as a Kaplan-Meyer curve, which is basically a time line, a graphical representation of the data over the course of time, or whether it should be presented as a cumulative type of summary table.

The data that were being reviewed with the VIGOR trial, again, it was an active control trial. The only comparator was naproxen. There were other data that the agency had reviewed from placebo controlled trials that were of similar length to the VIGOR trial that did not seem to be showing the cardiovascular finding at that time. So it was a complex discussion of analyzing the data and deciding how best to represent the data.

Mr. WAXMAN. Do you think anybody had in mind by a statement that would say that there is some uncertainty, but on the long-term impacts, that could be then used to muddy up the whole presentation to doctors, that, sort of like the tobacco companies used to do, it's not clear that the science indicates you are going to get all these diseases.

Dr. JENKINS. Right.

Chairman TOM DAVIS. The gentleman's time has expired. I will permit you to answer it.

Dr. JENKINS. Yes, that phraseology appears frequently in FDA-approved labeling, because we often cannot definitively conclude from the data that in fact the risk does accrue or in fact an individual patient will achieve that risk. But we present the information and then put that phraseology in to let people know that we have not definitively concluded about that issue.

Mr. WAXMAN. Thank you, Mr. Chairman.

Chairman TOM DAVIS. Thank you very much. Mr. Souder.

Mr. SOUDER. First I would like to ask unanimous consent to put my opening statement into the record.

Chairman TOM DAVIS. Without objection, so ordered.

[The prepared statement of Hon. Mark E. Souder follows:]

Statement of Congressman Mark Souder (R-IN)
Chairman, Subcommittee on Criminal Justice, Drug Policy and Human Resources
House Government Reform Committee
"Risk and Responsibility: The Roles of the FDA and Pharmaceutical Companies in
Ensuring the Safety of Approved Drugs, Like Vioxx"
May 5, 2005 10:00am
Washington, D.C.

The particular thrust of this hearing is to examine how the FDA and the drug manufacturer Merck handled the marketing, and ultimately the withdrawal, of Vioxx. The underlying issue in this situation, however, is much larger: *do we have an effective postmarketing safety program for approved drugs?*

In the face of criticism of the FDA and its handling of the Vioxx situation, the agency has publicly committed to taking certain steps for strengthening the safety program for marketed drugs. I hope we will hear from FDA's representative Dr. Galson specific ways the agency is addressing this issue.

Because drugs are being approved at a faster rate than ever, the result is that adverse problems may not become apparent until after the marketing process has begun. The early detection of serious adverse drug reactions has shifted from the pre-approval process, to the postmarketing phase.

Although companies themselves continue to study their drug after FDA approval—as Merck did for Vioxx—there is most likely a large gap between information that a pharmaceutical company may have, and information available to patients and physicians.

Therefore, detecting uncommon serious adverse drug events in marketed drugs under the current FDA system can be very difficult. This is a passive system reliant on voluntary reporting, and the data is frequently incomplete or insufficient.

Among proposals from outside the FDA to reform the safety programs for marketed drugs is a proposal to completely separate the drug approval process from the postmarketing safety and surveillance system. In other words, separate the Office of New Drugs (OND) from the Office of Drug Safety (OSD), in order to address the conflict inherent in trying to effectively monitor the safety of drugs that the same office just approved as safe for marketing.

Perhaps it is also worthwhile to consider whether or not an independent body that reviews and analyzes postmarketing data would be more effective than the current system that relies upon the data made available by the drug companies themselves.

This is a quote from the Journal of the American Medical Association (December 2004):

"The postmarketing surveillance system requires a long overdue major restructuring. Until that occurs…as epitomized by recent evidence of serious harms from widely used and heavily promoted medications, as demonstrated by the influence of industry over postmarketing data, and as illustrated by the lengths to which some manufacturers will go to protect their interests – the United States will still be far short of having an effective vigilant, and trustworthy system of postmarketing surveillance to protect the public."

I think today's hearing will shine a light on the problems that are inherent with the current postmarketing surveillance system, and I look forward to the testimony of all of today's witnesses.

Mr. SOUDER. I have a cluster of four different sets of questions that I am going to go through first. If you need to take notes, that's fine, or if I need to review it. They are all basically around the same category, which is post-marketing, for the most part, and studies related to post-marketing.

The companies continue to study these drugs afterwards, partly because of legal liabilities, partly for internal information. We rely on a passive system of reporting. Are there legal penalties imposed upon companies that withhold or conceal data, including data from any studies conducted before or after drug approval? That's one.

No. 2, there was already concern about cardiovascular risks on Cox–2 inhibitors as early as February 2001 from the FDA Arthritis Advisory Committee. Does the FDA—this is kind of a followup to what Mr. Towns asked earlier, and you clearly stated in your opening statement, and in your answer to him you said you could negotiate these things. In your opening statement you said that you could take definitive action.

My question is, do you have the authority to mandate a trial where it is apparent that such a trial would provide essential perspective information such as the incidence of cardiovascular events and possible association with Cox–2 treatment? If you have that power, as you suggested you might, definitive action would suggest you might, if you need to define definitive action further, why didn't you do it in this case, given the fact that your advisory council was already giving you some warning in the arthritis group?

The third area is that, if you allow data, if you are passive, in other words, if the companies are not mandated to give you this, and if you are not initiating a study, how do you see not only with Cox–2, but in the case of Oxycontin, for example, where there are all sorts of side effects that are developing, how do you take this into account? Isn't it possible that post-market reviews of this drug might have revealed a dangerous trend on Oxycontin long before it was made public? Is agency vigilance being turned over to the companies at the expense of identifying these trends early enough to stem larger problems?

Then last, and this is more directly to Dr. Jenkins and Dr. Seligman, although all of them kind of relate, we have had some concerns whether the Office of New Drugs and the Office of Drug Safety are communicating with each other. Could you tell us what you are doing to make sure that these two are cooperating and communicating better with each other? And specifically in the Office of Drug Safety, how is it getting more involved with both pre-approval and post-approval of drugs?

Dr. GALSON. Let me be the gatekeeper to help direct the questions. On the first one, I think very, very straight forwardly, companies are required to tell us about adverse events that they are aware of, and adverse information relating to their drugs, regardless of where it comes from, how it is collected. Does that answer that part?

Mr. SOUDER. Any penalties?

Dr. GALSON. Yes. Legal penalties. I don't know what they are at my fingertips.

Mr. SOUDER. Could you provide the committee what those are?

Dr. GALSON. Absolutely.

Dr. Jenkins, do you want to address the second one about the post-marketing authority, having to do with studies and Vioxx?

Dr. JENKINS. Specifically for Vioxx, you are describing the situation we were in in 2001 when we had the VIGOR trial, which showed a signal for cardiovascular risk, and you are asking, why didn't we require them to do another study to try to more definitively pin that down.

We thought about what the options were to try to get that information. There are some technical and practical considerations that come into play about trying to do a long-term study in patients with arthritis where you would use a placebo. Most patients are not going to want to be on placebo for long periods of time. So you get into practical questions.

We were aware that the sponsor was already conducting several very large studies looking at Vioxx for other indications, such as prevention of colon polyps and prevention of Alzheimer's disease. Those were situations where a placebo control was ethical and practical. We chose to focus our attention to working with the sponsor to assure that those studies were designed and adjudicated in a way that we could get information about the cardiovascular outcomes. And in fact the approved study that led to the withdrawal of Vioxx last September was just one of those studies, where we got the cardiovascular information from that placebo controlled setting.

Chairman TOM DAVIS. The gentleman's time has expired.

Is there anyone else who needs to answer that?

Mr. SOUDER. There was a third and fourth question.

Chairman TOM DAVIS. OK, you can finish answering.

Dr. GALSON. OK, quickly on the third, I think you are aware that we have been involved in making regulatory changes related to Oxycontin, because of our concerns from very early in the marketing, including promotional prosecution of the company, having to do with their promotion, and also changes in the labeling to reduce the chance of abuse of the drug, including working with a cross-agency group around the Government and within HHS. We are going to continue a high level of vigilance on this product and similar products because of the abuse concerns.

The last question I would like to have Dr. Seligman address.

Dr. SELIGMAN. Sure. In this last fiscal year, the Office of Drug Safety completed over 1,300 reviews and reports. The majority of these reviews that affect the pre- and post-market safety of a drug product were requested by and directed toward the Office of New Drugs. Clearly, communication is vital between the Office of Drug Safety and the 15 review divisions in that organization. We currently have a team from the Office of New Drugs and the Office of Drug Safety looking at ways to further enhance our regular communications.

But these reviews are only part of the daily sort of face to face interactions between our staff and a variety of venues to discuss and resolve safety issues. Recognizing the thousands of drugs that we monitor, the hundreds of issues that come up before us on a regular basis, it should not come as any surprise to you or the members of the committee that on occasion, either communications are not ideal or that communications may break down.

But we are committed on both sides to ensure that there is ongoing, effective, regular communication and that we work to resolve fairly and expeditiously any problems that may arise.

Chairman TOM DAVIS. Thank you very much. Mr. Kucinich.

Mr. KUCINICH. I thank the gentleman, and I thank the Chair and the ranking member for this hearing.

Now, it is interesting to hear the FDA's response, but when we are talking about Vioxx, Merck has displayed a litany of predatory behavior. We know from the record that Vioxx research teams were stacked with people who had financial associations with Merck, Merck manipulated research protocols. You know that they delayed publication of negative findings about Vioxx. They succeeded in getting people to take Vioxx that did not have medical need by spending $161 million for direct to consumer advertising alone and direct lobbying to doctors was a well-known practice that had the same result.

And last, you had 10 members of a 32-member FDA advisory board in charge of determining whether Vioxx should continue to be allowed on the market, they had ties to the industry. Had those advisors abstained, the committee would have voted that Vioxx should not have been returned to the market. And these are just the things we know about and there are other concerns that I am sure are going to be coming up as we dig deeper.

But what I am interested to know is this. With respect to the FDA's enforcement powers, if you see as we see in this case of Merck, where they had sales personnel going to doctors and giving them information which they knew to be false, which they told their doctors that, only to gain their own profit, why should the FDA even permit Merck to be in business? What have you done to provide discipline to protect the American consumers from drug companies who unscrupulously will continue the promotion of a product long after the questions of safety have been addressed and effectively discounted with respect to Vioxx?

Dr. GALSON. We have strong regulatory tools that we can use and that we do use to enforce our promotion regulations. Companies are not allowed to provide false or misleading information to physicians or consumers. We send them letters and warnings and additional regulatory action and fines when they do not follow the rules.

Mr. KUCINICH. But wait a minute. People are dying as a result of this. This isn't just a, well, you shouldn't do that again.

Dr. GALSON. Right.

Mr. KUCINICH. They were understating the incidence of cardiovascular mortality to doctors as a marketing tool. Have you ever, has the FDA ever contemplated telling Merck, you can't sell your drugs any more, that this is an offense against the public interest that is so powerful that you should not be permitted to stay in business?

Dr. GALSON. We really think the key to this is getting accurate information early to health care practitioners and patients, so that they do not have to just rely on the information from one source. We want them to hear from us what the latest information is about drugs, so that they can make their decisions with their physicians about whether——

Mr. KUCINICH. I don't know if you are hearing, with all due respect, I don't know if you are hearing my question. Maybe you are not the person to answer the question. But if you are not, maybe somebody in this room knows the answer to it. Does the FDA have the power to shut down a drug company that deliberately sold drugs that killed people?

Dr. GALSON. I think your question has many, many parts. The first, we prohibit people, companies from selling unsafe drugs. So yes, we have the capacity to stop a company from selling a drug that is unsafe. The assessment of whether a drug is unsafe is obviously very complex. In the Vioxx case, please keep in mind that an advisory committee that met in 2001 that included people from around the country who were experts in this gave us the advice that the risk-benefit profile of this drug was sufficient to allow it to stay on the market. So this is the advice that we were getting in 2001 from people who knew about those studies.

Mr. KUCINICH. And isn't it true that people on that advisory board had ties to the drug industry?

Dr. GALSON. I do not think that the ties or not ties or connections with the industry impacted the quality of the advice that we got. In any case, we make the final decision, not the advisory committee. Federal employees who have no ties to the drug industry.

Mr. KUCINICH. Do you personally take any kind of responsibility in what happens to American consumers as a result of the FDA not being strong enough in dealing with these companies?

Chairman TOM DAVIS. The gentleman's time has expired. If you want to answer that, you can.

Dr. GALSON. Of course I do, as do all the other 2000 incredibly dedicated people in the Drug Center.

Chairman TOM DAVIS. Thank you very much. This will end the questioning and I will dismiss this panel. We have two votes over on the House floor. When we come back, we will go with our second panel.

I want to thank all of you for being here and answering these questions.

We are in recess.

[The prepared statement of Hon. Dennis J. Kucinich follows:]

Statement of Dennis Kucinich
U.S. House of Representatives
Committee on Government Reform

Hearing: "Risk and Responsibility: The Roles of FDA and
Pharmaceutical Companies in Ensuring the Safety of
Approved Drugs Like Vioxx"
May 5, 2005

Thank you for the opportunity to speak, Chairman Davis about this critical public health issue that has affected the entire US. The Vioxx case presents us with a valuable opportunity to examine an industry in order to help it improve. The problem is not only that the FDA does not have sufficient regulatory authority to protect the public, though that is certainly true. The problem actually lies with the way pharmaceuticals are priced. I'll explain.

In the Vioxx case, Merck displayed a litany of predatory behavior. Vioxx research teams were stacked with people who had financial associations with Merck.[1] Merck manipulated research protocols.[2] They delayed publication of negative findings about Vioxx.[3] They succeeded in getting people to take Vioxx that did not have a medical need by spending $161 million[4] for direct-to-consumer advertising alone.[5] And direct lobbying to doctors is a well-

---

[1] See, for example, "Comparison of Upper GI Toxicity of Recoxefib and Naproxen in Patients with Rheumatoid Arthritis" in the 2000 New England Journal of Medicine where 11 of 13 authors have had financial associations with Merck and the other two are Merck employees. See also conflict of interest statements in "The Coxibs, Selective Inhibitors of Cyclooxygenase-2," New England Journal of Medicine, August 9, 2001. See also "Recommendations for the Medical Management of Osteoarthritis of the Hip and Knee" in Arthritis and Rheumatism, September 2000. There are several ties to Merck in each

[2] "A Nov. 21, 1996, memo by a Merck official shows…[Merck] wanted to conduct a trial to prove Vioxx was gentler on the stomach than older painkillers. But to show the difference most clearly, the Vioxx patients couldn't take any aspirin. In such a trial, 'there is a substantial chance that significantly higher rates' of cardiovascular problems would be seen in the Vioxx group, the memo said." And Alise Reicin, now a Merck vice president for clinical research "proposed that people with high risk of cardiovascular problems be kept out of the study so the difference in the rate of cardiovascular problems between the Vioxx patients and the others 'would not be evident.'"- Wall Street Journal, November 1, 2004

[3] Merck mentioned the ADVATAGE study at a 2001 conference but did not publish the results of the trial, which indicated that Vioxx users had a higher risk of heart attacks, until 2003.

[4] http://www.usatoday.com/news/health/2005-01-23-vioxx-usat_x.htm

[5] "The use of Cox-2 inhibitors skyrocketed from the time Vioxx hit the market in 1999. But now researchers have found that this rise occurred largely in patients who had little risk of developing a bleeding stomach ulcer. 'We found a rapid nationwide shift away from older, inexpensive drugs with better

known practice that has the same result. Lastly, ten members of 32 member FDA advisory board in charge of determining whether Vioxx should continue to be allowed on the market, had ties to industry. Had those advisers abstained, the committee would have voted that Vioxx should not return to the market.[6] And these are only the things we know about. More concerns are likely to be uncovered as we dig deeper.

Would Merck be doing all this if Merck was the only maker of Vioxx? Absolutely not. When there is competition in manufacturing, just like there is in most other sectors, the capability to squeeze so much profit from a single drug is gone. But under a monopoly, which is what Merck has with its patented Vioxx, the sky is the limit on profits. Only the patent holder or licensee can sell it, so they control the market. And when a company controls the market, they have considerable leeway to corrupt the process in ways similar to what we have seen with Merck.

The usual justification for patent monopolies is that patents are yielding innovation, which is critical for new pharmaceuticals. But we are not getting that innovation. The number of New Molecular Entities approved by the FDA has been in decline several years running. Copycats or me-too's constitute roughly 70% of new FDA approved drugs. In other words, the pipeline is drying up.

If we want to avoid another Vioxx down the road, we need to get to the root of the problem. We need to bring innovation back up, control perverse incentives, and drive drug prices back down to a similar level as other developed nations. We do that by changing the financing of pharmaceuticals.

Put simply, the NIH, which is currently responsible for much of the innovation in pharmaceutical research, should drastically increase its already successful pharmaceutical research program. The innovations that result should be available for any qualified entity to manufacture, which would introduce competition into the market. It would boost innovation, competition would drive down prices as it does in the generics market, and the incentive to engage in Merck-like behavior would be drastically reduced.

---

established safety and efficacy to newer, costly drugs with no real history.'"
http://my.webmd.com/content/Article/99/105308.htm?printing=true
[6] "10 Voters on Panel Backing Pain Pills Had Industry Ties,", New York Times, 2-2-05

[Recess.]

Chairman TOM DAVIS. Thank you all very much for being here. We are going to recognize our second and last panel. It will be Dr. Dennis Erb, vice president of global strategic regulatory development at Merck and Co. Doctor, thank you. Just to reiterate again, Merck is here voluntarily today, and we appreciate your being here. Dr. John Calfee, who is a resident scholar of the American Enterprise Institute, thank you for being with us. And Dr. Michael Wilkes, the vice dean for medical education, at the School of Medicine, University of California at Davis.

It is our committee's policy that we swear in witnesses before you testify, so if you will just rise with me and raise your right hands.

[Witnesses sworn.]

Chairman TOM DAVIS. Thank you.

The rules are, your entire written testimony is on the record. This is being televised, though, and I know particularly, Dr. Erb, we have had some comments about the company. I want to give you ample time, if you need more than 5 minutes, to lay out anything you need to lay out. We are going to start the questioning with 10 minutes with me and 10 with Mr. Waxman and then go to Members. That's by agreement of Mr. Waxman and myself.

So thanks again. Again, I will just reiterate, you are appearing here voluntarily. We appreciate that, and you're on.

STATEMENTS OF DENNIS ERB, PH.D., VICE PRESIDENT OF GLOBAL STRATEGIC REGULATORY DEVELOPMENT, MERCK AND CO., INC.; JOHN E. CALFEE, RESIDENT SCHOLAR, AMERICAN ENTERPRISE INSTITUTE; MICHAEL WILKES, VICE DEAN FOR MEDICAL EDUCATION, SCHOOL OF MEDICINE, UNIVERSITY OF CALIFORNIA, DAVIS

STATEMENT OF DENNIS ERB, PH.D.

Mr. ERB. Thank you. I just have some opening comments.

Mr. Chairman, Congressman Waxman, members of the committee, my name is Dennis Erb. I am responsible for Merck's interactions with pharmaceutical regulatory agencies around the world, including the U.S. FDA. I am pleased to be able to discuss with you the important issues of the safety of FDA-approved drugs.

We appreciate the committee's attention in this important matter. I hope that today by discussing with you Merck's actions to study Vioxx following its approval we can assist the committee in understanding the role of post-approval clinical trials. It was through such trials that Merck diligently pursued information to further clarify the benefits and risks of Vioxx.

Our original application to the FDA for Vioxx included data from many studies involving approximately 10,000 patients. These studies compared the effects of Vioxx to other non-steroidal anti-inflammatory medicines, or NSAIDs, and to placebo, and included studies of patients who had been on Vioxx for longer than 1 year. The FDA, as well as an independent advisory panel, agreed that Vioxx was safe and effective when used in accordance with its prescribing information. FDA approved Vioxx in May 1999.

Once approved, we continued to study Vioxx. Consistent with our history of scientific excellence, Merck initiated long-term post-approval trials to investigate new uses for Vioxx and to further clarify its safety profile. We conducted many large post-approval trials for Vioxx with extensive input from the FDA. In fact, since submitting its original application, Merck has completed approximately 70 trials on Vioxx, involving more than 40,000 patients.

In one of those large trials, known as VIGOR, there was a higher incidence in cardiovascular thrombotic events in patients taking Vioxx compared to the NSAID naproxen. This result stood in contrast to our other data on Vioxx. In a pooled analysis of clinical trials submitted for the FDA approval, there were similar rates of cardiovascular thrombotic events between Vioxx and placebo and between Vioxx and NSAIDs other than naproxen.

Further, in two large ongoing placebo-controlled trials, we found no difference in the rates of cardiovascular thrombotic events between Vioxx and placebo. These data led us to conclude that the difference in cardiovascular event rates in the VIGOR resulted from the anti-platelet effect of naproxen.

We promptly disclosed the results of this clinical trial and our interpretation of it to the FDA, physicians, the scientific community and the media. The cardiovascular results of VIGOR were widely reported and discussed at the time. We worked diligently with FDA to review the data and develop revised prescribing information. We also recognized the value and interest in obtaining additional cardiovascular safety data on Vioxx. We undertook additional clinical trials to do so.

We believed wholeheartedly in the safety of Vioxx and that Vioxx was an important treatment option for physicians and their patients. The labeling for NSAIDs has for a number of years included a warning about serious and potentially fatal gastrointestinal events. Vioxx was the only approved NSAID demonstrated to reduce the risk of serious gastrointestinal side effects, compared to those on other NSAIDs.

This was an important benefit for many who suffered from the pain of arthritis and other conditions. On a personal level, I believe in the value that Vioxx provided to patients. My own father was taking Vioxx until we voluntarily withdrew it from the marketplace.

Mr. Chairman, in the 7-months since that withdrawal, there have been many questions and much discussion about the evidence of the safety of Vioxx. Yet while Vioxx was on the market, in the combined analysis of our controlled clinical trials, there was no demonstrated increased risk of cardiovascular or thrombotic events for patients taking Vioxx compared to patients taking placebo or NSAIDs other than naproxen. Merck continued to conduct post-approval trials of Vioxx. In one of those, the APPROVe trial, there was an increased risk of confirmed cardiovascular events beginning after 18 months of continuous daily treatment in patients taking Vioxx compared to those taking placebo.

Given the questions raised by the data and the availability of alternative therapies, we decided that withdrawing the medicine was the responsible course to take. Today, Mr. Chairman, we know that the science has continued to evolve, and new data on some of the alternative therapies to Vioxx have become available. This data was publicly reviewed by a special advisory committee in February.

Both the committee and the FDA have concluded that the increased cardiovascular risks seen in the APPROVe trial is shared by other Cox–2 inhibitors.

FDA also concluded that all NSAIDs should have a cardiovascular risk warning. Given the unique benefits of Vioxx, Merck is considering this new data and will discuss their implications for Vioxx with the FDA and other regulatory authorities around the world.

In conclusion, Mr. Chairman, throughout Merck's history, it has been our rigorous adherence to scientific investigation, openness and integrity that has enabled us to bring new medicines to the people who need them. We believe Merck acted appropriately and responsibly to extensively study Vioxx after it was approved for marketing to gain more clinical information about the medicine, and we promptly disclosed the results of these studies to FDA, physicians, the scientific community, and the media.

I will be pleased to respond to your questions.

[The prepared statement of Mr. Erb follows:]

Testimony of Dennis Erb, Ph.D.
Vice President, Global Strategic Regulatory Development
Merck & Co., Inc
before the Committee on Government Reform
United States House of Representatives
May 5, 2005

Mr. Chairman, Congressman Waxman, members of the Committee, I am Dennis Erb. I am responsible for Merck's interactions with pharmaceutical regulatory agencies around the world including the U.S. FDA. I am pleased to be able to discuss with you the important issue of the safety of FDA-approved drugs.

We appreciate the Committee's attention to this important matter. I hope that today, by discussing with you Merck's actions to study Vioxx following its approval, we can assist the Committee in understanding the role of post-approval clinical trials. It was through such trials that Merck diligently pursued information to further clarify the benefits and risks of Vioxx.

Our original application to the FDA for Vioxx included data from many studies involving approximately 10,000 patients. These studies compared the effects of Vioxx to other nonsteroidal anti-inflammatory medicines or NSAIDs and to placebo and included studies of patients who had been on Vioxx for longer than one year. The FDA and an independent advisory panel agreed that Vioxx was safe and effective when used in accordance with its prescribing information. FDA approved Vioxx in May of 1999.

Once approved, we continued to study Vioxx. Consistent with our history of scientific excellence, Merck initiated long-term, post-approval trials to investigate new uses for Vioxx and to further clarify its safety profile. We conducted many, large, post-approval trials for Vioxx with extensive input from the FDA. In fact, since submitting its original application, Merck has completed approximately 70 clinical trials on Vioxx involving more than 40,000 patients.

In one of those large trials – known as VIGOR – there was a higher incidence of cardiovascular thrombotic events in patients taking Vioxx compared to the NSAID naproxen. This result stood in contrast to our other data on Vioxx. In a pooled analysis of the clinical trials submitted for FDA approval, there were similar rates of cardiovascular thrombotic events between Vioxx and placebo, and between Vioxx and NSAIDs other than naproxen. Further, in two large on-going placebo-controlled trials, we found no difference in the rates of cardiovascular thrombotic events between Vioxx and placebo. These data led us to conclude that the difference in the cardiovascular event rates in VIGOR resulted from the anti-platelet effect of naproxen.

We promptly disclosed the results of this clinical trial and our interpretation of it to the FDA, physicians, the scientific community and the media. The cardiovascular results of VIGOR were widely reported and discussed at the time. We worked diligently with the FDA to review the data and develop revised prescribing information. And we also recognized the value and interest in obtaining additional cardiovascular safety data on Vioxx and we undertook additional clinical trials to do so.

We believed wholeheartedly in the safety of Vioxx and that Vioxx was an important treatment option for physicians and their patients. The labeling for NSAIDs has, for a number of years, included a warning about serious, and potentially fatal, gastrointestinal events. Vioxx was the only approved NSAID demonstrated to reduce the risk of serious gastrointestinal side effects compared to those on other NSAIDs. This was an important benefit for many who suffered from the pain of arthritis and other conditions.

On a personal level, I believed in the value that Vioxx provided to patients. My own father was a regular user of Vioxx until we voluntarily withdrew it from the market.

Mr. Chairman, in the seven months since that withdrawal, there have been many questions, and much discussion about the evidence of the safety of Vioxx. Yet, while Vioxx was on the market, the combined analysis of our controlled clinical trials demonstrated no increased risk of cardiovascular thrombotic events for patients taking Vioxx compared to patients taking placebo or NSAIDs other than naproxen.

Merck continued to conduct post-approval trials of Vioxx. In one of those – the APPROVe trial – there was an increased risk of confirmed cardiovascular events beginning after 18 months of continuous daily treatment in patients taking Vioxx compared to those taking placebo. Given the questions raised by the data and the availability of alternative therapies, we decided that withdrawing the medicine was the responsible course to take.

Today, Mr. Chairman, we know that the science has continued to evolve and new data on some of the alternative therapies to Vioxx have become available. These data were publicly reviewed by a special Advisory Committee in February. Both that Committee and the FDA have concluded that the increased cardiovascular risk seen in the APPROVe trial is shared by other COX-2 inhibitors. FDA also concluded that all NSAIDs should have a cardiovascular risk warning.

Given the unique benefits of Vioxx, Merck is considering these new data and will discuss their implications for Vioxx with the FDA and other regulatory authorities around the world.

In conclusion, Mr. Chairman, throughout Merck's history, it has been our rigorous adherence to scientific investigation, openness and integrity that has enabled us to bring new medicines to people who need them. We believe Merck acted appropriately and responsibly to extensively study Vioxx after it was approved for marketing to gain more clinical information about the medicine. And we promptly disclosed the results of these studies to the FDA, physicians, the scientific community and the media.

I will be pleased to respond to your questions.

Chairman TOM DAVIS. Thank you very much, Dr. Erb.

Mr. Calfee? I guess it is Dr. Calfee, a doctor from Berkeley, CA, too, Mr. Waxman.

STATEMENT OF JOHN E. CALFEE, PH.D.

Mr. CALFEE. Thank you for inviting me to testify. It is an honor to be here. I would like to briefly summarize four points from the written statement I submitted for the record.

First, I think the FDA is doing a reasonably good job of drug safety surveillance, but it can do better, and probably will do better in the near future. We must recognize that drug safety monitoring is difficult to do well. Our healthcare system is highly decentralized, liability of fear inhibits full and frank reporting. Patients often see more than one physician and often take over-the-counter drugs without their physician's knowledge. When something goes wrong, it is not easy to distinguish between inherent drug safety and other factors, including mis-prescribing, patient noncompliance, medical error, and the imperfect nature of many widely used drug therapies.

The FDA's recent drug initiatives may substantially improve drug safety, but this is by no means certain. I would caution Congress, however, against creating an independent drug safety board with the power to overrule FDA staff decisions. Such a board would impede one of the FDA's most essential tasks, which is the everyday balancing of the costs and benefits of recently approved drugs as new information flows in from the field. The creation of a separate group dedicated only to safety raises the dangerous prospect of failing to give proper weight to keeping useful drugs on the market unburdened by overly alarmist warnings.

Second, I strongly disagree with critics about what Merck should have done after the VIGOR trial was concluded in 2000. Although that trial revealed an excess of adverse cardiovascular events compared to naproxen, it was far from clear that Vioxx was a unique problem. Very little was known about the real issue, which was whether non-selective NSAIDs in general, and naproxen in particular, were beneficial, harmful or neutral in their cardiovascular effects. Forcing patients to switch to another NSAID could have done more harm than good, especially for those at risk for ulcers.

I also take issue with the idea that Merck should have undertaken a large long-term clinical trial devoted to Vioxx's cardiovascular side effects. Given the mystery surrounding NSAIDs generally, it made little sense to focus exclusively on Vioxx. I refer here to placebo-controlled studies. The fact that Merck actually began a large placebo-controlled cancer prevention trial that included cardiovascular end points was sufficient in these circumstances.

A final issue is direct to consumer advertising. There is little evidence that DTC advertising played a crucial role in either the growth of the Cox–2 market or the expansion of that market beyond patients who are demonstrably at high risk for ulcers. In fact, similar trends occurred in other nations, such as Australia, where DTC advertising was prohibited.

Third, I think that for the most part the FDA's refusal to undertake drastic action after 2000 was correct and that events had borne out the wisdom of their approach. I say this as a veteran critic of the FDA, but even I have to recognize that sometimes the FDA gets it right. The FDA instantly recognized that the issue was not Vioxx, but the entire NSAID class.

The ambiguous results of the 2000 VIGOR trial provided little reason to remove Vioxx from the market. Those results were thoroughly discussed in the medical literature, however, and were taken into account in the updated practice guides provided by leading professional physician organizations. This process was superior to either removing the drug or issuing alarming warnings more stringent than the one that was actually added to the Vioxx label.

As was explained in the insightful April 6, 2005 memo by FDA staffers John Jenkins and Paul Seligman, whom you heard from earlier today, the totality of the evidence provides no persuasive reason to think that Vioxx is more dangerous than other Cox–2s or that the Cox–2s as a class are more dangerous than traditional nonselective NSAIDs. This is the single most important message from this entire episode.

Fourth, and finally, a few words about the impact of the Vioxx episode on the FDA itself. The FDA is notorious among many economists for putting too much weight on safety when approving new drugs. That is inevitable, however, because the penalties for approving a new drug that turns out badly are far greater than the penalties for being too conservative in approving new drugs.

The Vioxx episode has reinforced that situation. The massive and unrestrained criticism visited on the FDA in the Vioxx episode greatly exceeds any criticism the agency has received in recent years for moving too slowly. The FDA has learned once again that it is better to be too careful than to expeditiously make innovative drugs available to patients.

The danger now is that the FDA will retreat even further, making the process of getting innovative drugs to market even more costly and time-consuming. Fortunately, the FDA has shown considerable courage in resisting outside pressure to make truly harmful decisions. I urge Congress not to make things worse by imposing penalties or unwise structural changes on this agency.

That concludes my oral remarks, Mr. Chairman.

[The prepared statement of Mr. Calfee follows:]

John E. Calfee, Ph.D.

American Enterprise Institute
1150 17th St., NW, Washington, D.C.
202-862-7175 -- fax 202-862-7177 -- email: calfeej@aei.org

Written testimony

Before the

United States House of Representatives

Committee on Government Reform

Public Hearings on

"The Roles of FDA and Pharmaceutical Companies in

Ensuring the Safety of Approved Drugs, Like Vioxx."

May 5, 2005

I am honored to testify in the May 5, 2005 House Government Reform hearings on "The Roles of FDA and Pharmaceutical Companies in Ensuring the Safety of Approved Drugs, Like Vioxx." I am a Resident Scholar at the American Enterprise Institute for Public Policy Research, where I have conducted research on pharmaceutical markets and other topics. The views I present are my own and do not necessarily represent those of the American Enterprise Institute. Much of this testimony draws on an unpublished article written by my colleague Ximena Pinell and me, which covers the Vioxx incident and its significance in considerable detail (Calfee and Pinell 2005).

1. FDA's Surveillance of Post-approval Drug Safety

Any assessment of post-approval drug safety surveillance must begin by acknowledging the extraordinary difficulty of that task. Our health care system is highly decentralized with thousands of individual physicians, clinics, and hospitals, most of which do not share data. Patients often receive care from more than one organization, and they self-administer over-the-counter (OTC) drugs, many of which compete directly with powerful prescription drugs. The tort liability system undermines incentives of physicians and others to report in a timely and forthright manner events that might involve drug safety but might also involve error or perceived error (Leape 2002). Finally, many adverse drug events carry ambiguous implications because of the difficulty of separating inherent drug safety from patient misuse, physician error, hospital error, and above all, the difficulty of administering many drugs–including such common drugs as insulin, heparin, and warfarin–which are both very useful and very dangerous (Gurwitz, et al. 2003). The pervasive problems in monitoring the safety of drugs or indeed the safety of any important component of health care have been widely recognized (Bates 1998; Leape 2002).

The FDA appears to recognize these problems and seems eager to address them by encouraging better record-keeping and communication in the health care system, more efficient methods for reporting potential problems to the FDA, increased attention to safety during pre-market testing, and enhanced post-approval monitoring. In March 2005, the FDA issued a series of guidances for the pharmaceutical industry on pre-market risk assessment, post-approval monitoring, and pharmacovigilance (the surveillance of side-effects) and pharmacoepidemiology (the study of a drug's efficacy and safety using large data sets) (FDA 2005a, b, c, d). These initiatives address two fundamental components of drug safety: how drugs work in clinical practice, and how to communicate drug safety information and practices to physicians and patients.

The process of communicating about drug safety is fraught with difficulties such as over-warning and consequent under-use of valuable drugs. This was pointed out in a 2003 speech by former FDA Commissioner Mark McClellan. After describing a litigant's attempt to add a suicide warning to an antidepressant drug's label despite the FDA's rejection of it three times on scientific grounds, McClellan warned, "the drawing of unwarranted attention to an unproven but serious risk could lead to undertreatment of depression." The problem is also widely appreciated in the medical community. An example is the American Psychiatric Association's strong opposition to the "black box" warning added to the labels of popular antidepressants, which, by deterring their use, "would put seriously ill patients at grave risk" (APA press release 2004).

It is unlikely that the FDA now performs these difficult tasks as well as they can be done. On the other hand, clear paths to unambiguous improvement are not well established. Although I would be the last person to argue that the FDA does its overall job in an unimpeachable manner, I would nonetheless warn against forcing the FDA into abrupt changes in its handling of the safety of approved drugs. In particular, the creation of an independent drug safety board insulated from the FDA's drug approval and oversight staff would severely hamper the already difficult task of balancing the costs and benefits of new drugs (for reasons discussed below).

2. The Cox-2 class of NSAIDs

Merck's Vioxx (rofecoxib) is a member of the class of drugs known as Cox-2 inhibitors. The Cox-2s are part of the larger class of NSAIDs (non-steroidal anti-inflammatory drugs), which includes such popular pain relievers as Alleve (naproxen), Advil (ibuprofen), and several prescription-only drugs, along with the original NSAID, aspirin. The traditional NSAIDs are probably the most-used of any drug category worldwide, especially for treating arthritis pain, but they often cause upper gastro-intestinal (G.I.) ulcers and bleeding. This can cause pain and even death. The most reliable estimate of the death toll from NSAID use in the United States is between ten and twenty thousand deaths annually (Wolfe, Lichtenstein, and Singh 1999).

The Cox-2s were developed after researchers discovered some fifteen years ago that NSAIDs suppressed both the Cox-1 enzyme, which is protective of the stomach and the rest of the G.I. system, and the Cox-2 enzyme, which reinforces inflammation and thus causes pain. This insight suggested that if research firms could develop selective NSAIDs, which suppress mainly the Cox-2 enzyme, those drugs could offer pain relief with less G.I. harm. The arrival of the first Cox-2 inhibitors, Celebrex (celecoxib; Pfizer) and Vioxx, was greeted with enthusiasm by the medical community, especially those who treat arthritis: "That these COX-2 selective inhibitors have become so successful within the same year of their launch attests to the perceived need for novel agents that can control the signs and symptoms of inflammatory diseases, but with minimal risk of gastrointestinal side effects" (Whittle 2000).

It turned out that the Cox-2 enzyme is implicated in cancer as well as inflammation, which opened a line of research into the Cox-2 inhibitors as cancer preventives or treatments (Chau and Cunningham 2002). Also, inflammation has been identified as important in conditions other arthritis, including Alzheimer's and coronary heart disease. Hence pharmaceutical firms pursued numerous clinical trials on cancer prevention and other illnesses as well as on arthritis treatment.

On September 30, 2004, Merck withdrew Vioxx from the market without consulting with the FDA after results from a nearly completed three-year clinical trial in cancer prevention revealed a statistically significant increase in heart attacks and other adverse cardiovascular events such as strokes (Bresalier 2005). Merck took this action because it believed that Vioxx was unique among the Cox-2 inhibitor class of drugs in its cardiovascular risk profile (Merck 2004).

A storm of criticism descended upon both Merck and the FDA for not having taken various actions—including the withdrawal of Vioxx—months or years earlier (e.g., Topol 2004; *Lancet*, Dec. 4, 2004). Critics included leading medical journals and academic medical researchers, newspaper editorials and op-ed writers, and participants in Congressional hearings. I believe that as events proceeded and research results were compiled, much of this criticism proved to be excessive if not unfounded.

3. What Should Merck Have Done Earlier?

A. Should Merck Have Conducted More Studies of Cardiovascular Risk?

The clinical trials that provided the foundation for FDA approval of Vioxx had revealed no excess cardiovascular problems in comparison to traditional NSAIDs. There were some signs of risk relative to placebos--i.e., relative to the use of no pain reliever at all--but as FDA staff noted at the time, this was true of all NSAIDs (Pelayo 1999). The large-scale VIGOR trial, published in November 2000 (more than a year after Vioxx was approved for marketing), revealed dramatically lower G.I. problems but unexpectedly showed a significantly higher level of heart attacks and strokes (Bombardier, et al., 2000). The implications of this result were far from clear. A substantial fraction (38 percent) of heart attacks was in patients for whom low-dose aspirin was indicated (due to history of heart attacks or other cardiovascular complications) but who failed to take it (the trial avoided accepting patients on aspirin). For other patients, heart attack rates did not differ significantly. Because heart attacks were not a pre-defined endpoint in the VIGOR trial, because Vioxx had been compared to naproxen, a traditional NSAID, rather than to a placebo, and because other trials involving both Vioxx and Celebrex had not revealed significant cardiovascular problems, it was by so means obvious that Vioxx would in fact cause excess heart attacks compared to placebos. Obvious alternatives were that the result was partly a statistical fluke (always possible when selecting a non-predefined endpoint for analysis) or that the comparator, naproxen, was instead cardio-protective. Subsequent research strongly suggested that naproxen is at least moderately cardio-protective (Dalen 2002; Juni, et al. 2004).

A natural question, raised in the medical literature and elsewhere (cf. Mukherjee, et al. 2001) was whether Merck should immediately mount another clinical trial, presumably against a placebo instead of another NSAID, in order learn with more certainty whether Vioxx causes heart attacks. But what trial to run? Considerable debate centered on what population to study: patients with high risk for heart attacks and strokes (whose comorbidities and multiple drug use would greatly complicate the trial), or some other population? Unless several large trials were launched, crucial questions would remain. Yet running even a single trial with sufficient power to detect a doubling of a small long-term risk would involve thousands of patients spread across scores or hundreds of medical practices, at a cost of tens of millions of dollars or more, and require one to three years for design, execution and analysis.

An equally important question was which drug to test. Vioxx was probably not the best target. As the FDA has repeatedly pointed out, traditional NSAIDs had never been subjected to large, long-term trials like VIGOR.[1] The fact that NSAIDs reduce inflammation, which is implicated in heart attacks, suggests that they could prevent heart attacks. But analysis of the biological mechanisms involved in NSAIDs generates ambiguous results, suggesting that Cox-2s and other NSAIDs could facilitate rather than impede the processes that lead to heart attacks (Fitzgerald 2001). As one researcher pointed out in *The Lancet*, the common observation that arthritis patients have more heart attacks has been seen as implicating arthritis itself; but it is impossible to rule out the possibility that the heart attack risk derives instead from the extremely common use of NSAIDs by arthritis patients (Scott and Watts 2005). Because most of what was already known about NSAIDs and cardiovascular disease had come from Cox-2 clinical trials, it probably made more sense to start work on traditional NSAIDs. This line of research would in fact be recommended by the FDA in its April 7, 2005 NSAID initiative (FDA press release April 7, 2005). Given the fact that none of the traditional NSAIDs are under patent, such trials would have to be sponsored by NIH or another public source.

It so happened that in 2001, Merck was already planning a large, placebo-controlled trial (called APPROVe) to test whether Vioxx could prevent colorectal cancer. By adding cardiovascular endpoints, the APPROVe trial could detect significant cardiovascular risk. Given these circumstances, it is hard to see why Merck had an obligation to do more than run the very expensive APPROVe trial with its cardiovascular

---

[1] *New York Times*, October 19, 2004: "Dr. Janet Woodcock, acting deputy commissioner for operations at the F.D.A., said in a speech at the American College of Rheumatology meeting in San Antonio yesterday that 'at this point we don't have any definitive evidence' that the COX-2 inhibitors as a class are more risky than older painkillers like ibuprofen and naproxen."

endpoints. Events have vindicated this view. The tight focus of academic and other critics on Vioxx and Merck proved misplaced. When the FDA issued its most definitive report on NSAIDs (Jenkins and Seligman 2005) and undertook a major initiative in the NSAID market on April 7, 2005, it made perfectly clear that what began as a Vioxx incident was in fact an NSAID issue. It stated that there is no convincing evidence that Vioxx is more dangerous than other Cox-2s in terms of cardiovascular risk or that Cox-2s as a class are more dangerous than traditional NSAIDs. The agency therefore required cardiovascular warnings for all NSAIDs and urged NIH and other agencies to undertake large-scale clinical trials of traditional NSAIDs (Jenkins and Seligman 2005; FDA press release Apr. 7, 2005).

B. Should Merck Have Curtailed or Redirected Consumer Advertising?

Another issue is Vioxx advertising, especially direct-to-consumer (DTC) advertising. Although commentators have often assumed that DTC advertising played a large role in the uptake of Cox-2s, this is far from clear from the factual record. Total Cox-2 DTC advertising in the year 2003 was $165 million (*New York Times* Dec. 21, 2004) compared to sales of $4.4 billion (IMS Health, IMS National Sales Perspectives). Such a small advertising-to-sales ratio suggests limited returns to advertising.

Also instructive is experience abroad. In Canada, the arrival of the first two Cox-2s, Celebrex and Vioxx, caused a 50 percent increase in NSAID prescribing (Mamdani, Rochon, Laupacis, and Anderson 2002). Vioxx was reportedly the fastest selling new drug in the history of the U.K. health system (Emery, Hawkey, and Moore 2001), although its sales remained small by U.S. standards. In Australia, the first two Cox-2s, Celebrex and Vioxx, gained sales so rapidly as to cause an immediate fiscal "calamity" in the government-subsidized drug benefit. None of these nations permit DTC advertising. As in the U.S., the rapid uptake of Cox-2s reflected the initial enthusiasm of medical experts and innate consumer preferences more than the force of advertising.

A related issue is whether Vioxx and competing Cox-2s were used primarily by patients at high risk for upper G.I. problems. In general, Cox-2 usage extended well beyond that group. This is partly because some patients encounter serious G.I. bleeding with little warning in their personal histories, as reflected in prominent practice guides that recommended Cox-2s as first-line arthritis pain therapies (American Pain Society 2002; American Geriatric Society 2002). But other factors essentially guaranteed broad usage. Vioxx and other Cox-2s offer simplified dosage (one or two pills a day instead of two or more pills several times a day), with less need to take additional drugs to prevent heartburn or ulcers. For some patients, a Cox-2 provides superior pain relief (reflecting individual differences in patient response to drug therapy). With most patients paying only a small co-payment, Cox-2s were clearly attractive to a broad range of users. Thus an early Australian study found that more than two-thirds of Cox-2 patients had not previously been prescribed a traditional NSAID, and up to 60 percent had not been prescribed *any* painkiller in the preceding year (Kerr, et al, 2003). A Canadian study of Cox-2 usage found only a moderate tendency toward patients at high G.I. risk despite a requirement that physicians document a G.I.-related need (Mamdani, Rochon, Laupacis, and Anderson 2002).

Oddly enough, advertising was strongly limited in its ability to target Cox-2 usage. DTC advertising was banned altogether in Canada and Australia, of course. But even in the U.S., FDA rules prohibited manufacturers from advertising the G.I. benefits of Cox-2s. Such benefits had not been documented (at least, not to the FDA's satisfaction) in the trials that supported FDA approval. G.I. protection was never on the FDA-approved Celebrex label, and even after the APPROVe trial, Merck still had to warn patients of G.I. risks because Vioxx had reduced, but did not entirely eliminate, G.I. complications. Thus neither consumer advertising nor promotion directed at physicians could easily target high G.I. risk patients.

4. What should the FDA have done earlier?

The common argument that the FDA should have moved rapidly to force Vioxx off the market or require vigorous warnings and/or large-scale clinical trials (e.g., Topol 2004; *Lancet*, Dec. 4, 2004) has proved largely unfounded. Consider the question of whether the FDA should have required a strong cardiovascular warning shortly after the VIGOR results were released in 2000. One should take into account the fact that the VIGOR results were widely discussed and debated in the medical community. Several Cox-2 and NSAID reviews published during this period (e.g., Dalen 2002; Bjarnason, Takeuchi, and Simpson 2003; and Whittle 2003) all reached roughly the same set of conclusions: The Cox-2s provided important G.I. protection. Most trials had not revealed significant cardiovascular problems, but at least one large trial (VIGOR) had. The VIGOR results might have been caused by a cardioprotective property of naproxen, but Vioxx itself might also have been the problem. Thus possible CVD side-effects should be monitored even as Cox-2s are prescribed for their original purpose of providing pain relief while reducing G.I. side-effects.[2] These ad hoc reviews were complemented by periodic updating of practice guidelines issued by professional organizations and practitioner-oriented journals (e.g., American Pain Society 2002; American Geriatric Society 2002; American College of Rheumatology treatment guidelines in Schnitzer 2002). It seems clear that the most important data on cardiovascular side-effects associated with Vioxx were widely disseminated and digested in the medical community. One indication of the market effects is the fact that after an extraordinarily rapid uptake in the first two years, Cox-2 sales were essentially flat in 2001 through 2004 (Calfee and Pinell 2005, table 1).

Given these circumstances, it seems unlikely that a quicker addition of a cardiovascular warning to the Vioxx label would have significantly improved medical practice. In fact, it might have impeded best practices; the FDA eventually concluded that even with the APPROVe results in hand, there is no compelling evidence that other Cox-2s or other NSAIDs are significantly safer than Vioxx in terms of adverse cardiovascular side-effects.

---

[2] Bjarnason, et al. 2003 noted, "The incidence of these [cardiovascular] side effects is very unlikely to outweigh the benefits of the improved gastrointestinal tolerability."

For much the same reason, it would have been a mistake for the FDA to have forced Vioxx off the market because of the VIGOR findings. Doing so would have pushed prescribing toward other Cox-2s or more likely, traditional NSAIDs. Again, there was little evidence at the time (and little evidence now) that this would have benefited patients.

I have already discussed the question of whether Merck should have conducted additional clinical trials to assess cardiovascular side-effects. The same reasoning applies here. Just as it made little sense to push forward with trials of Vioxx instead of other NSAIDs, the FDA had little reason to force Merck to launch such trials, especially in light of the fact that Merck was already preparing to start a cancer trial that would include cardiovascular endpoints.

5. Impact of the Vioxx episode on the FDA

The FDA has long been criticized by economists and others for being too cautious in approving new drugs. An excessive emphasis on safety is perfectly understandable given the incentives faced by FDA staff. If the staff is too slow to approve a new drug, almost no one notices because few people know enough to assess what patients have been losing. But if a drug gets approved and then runs into safety problems, public awareness is widespread and quickly expanded through the news media and other sources. If there is an institutional bias at the FDA, it is toward excessive emphasis on safety in approving new drugs and leaving them on the market, rather than a lax attitude toward safety.

Some FDA critics have cited the Vioxx withdrawal as evidence that even if the FDA has sometimes been too cautious, the situation has changed because a substantial proportion of FDA funding comes from industry user fees. The argument is that the FDA has gotten too close to the industry and therefore inappropriately discounts safety in order get drugs on the market sooner and keep them there (e.g., Topol 2004). Quite aside from the fact that the PDUFA law that mandates user fees simply requires the FDA to make decisions faster–but not to make decisions more favorable to the industry–it is clear from the Vioxx episode that the incentives for FDA staff to maintain at least reasonable drug safety standards--or even much higher standards--remains largely undisturbed. The fusillade of criticism directed at the agency over Vioxx and Cox-2s--especially from its most reliable base of support, the academic medical community and the most prestigious medical journals--vastly exceeds any criticism it has received in recent years for being too slow to approve new drugs or too quick to remove them.

Thus the Vioxx episode has probably made it more difficult for the FDA to do its job and has probably pushed the FDA even further than usual toward excessive caution in guiding manufacturers through clinical trials and the approval process. This is reflected partly in institutional changes such as the creation of Drug Safety Oversight Board that includes outside experts (FDA, February 15, 2005 Press release). This body is purely advisory and will not have authority to relabel or withdraw drugs. Whether it will reinforce the agency's natural tendency toward over-caution remains to be seen. But at least it is vastly superior to the creation of a fully independent board with power to remove drugs or change their labeling, as some have proposed to do through legislation (e.g., *Lancet*, Feb. 26, 2005). An independent board would necessarily impede the routine balancing of costs and benefits of drugs that must occur as post-approval data provides new information on both unexpected problems and surprisingly high (or low) efficacy. Nor would an independent board avoid be immune to having an interest in approved drugs. The board would necessarily make repeated rulings on the same drug in response to a series of safety alarms. This would leave board members with the same stake in their past decisions that the FDA's drug approval staff now have, but without an off-setting responsibility to assure that useful drugs remain available to physicians and patients.

The Vioxx episode appears to have led the FDA to take other measures that could prove harmful to the development and use of valuable new drugs. The agency has begun to require more warnings, especially the "black box" warnings that can dominate prescribing information (an example being the April 11 imposition of black box warnings on seven anti-psychotic drugs; *Wall Street Journal*, April 12, 2005). As was pointed out by professional physician organizations in connection with the required black box pediatric suicide warning for the SSRI class of antidepressants, too many warnings can cause as much harm as too few warnings, leading to under-use of drugs that treat or prevent conditions that are themselves dangerous (APA 2004). News reports suggest that is exactly what has happened (*New York Times*, September 16, 2004).

The FDA has also moved aggressively to make emerging results from clinical trials available to physicians and the general public via a Drug Watch Web Page (FDA, February 15, 2005 Press release). Although this initiative may seem harmless, it could end up yielding more costs than benefits. Undigested clinical trial results can be highly misleading in terms of apparent drug benefits as well as drug side-effects. The Drug Watch Web Page initiative therefore merits close scrutiny by anyone interested in drug development, drug therapy and drug safety. It could generate a variety of undesirable effects ranging from unjustified liability attacks and inappropriate switches to older (and less safe) drugs to unfounded promotional activities.

Finally, there is the strong possibility that the FDA is moving toward even greater caution in approving new drugs and in the requirements it imposes on the clinical trials necessary to gain marketing approval. Certainly, this prospect is being widely discussed in the drug development community.

References

American Geriatrics Society (2002) "The Management of Persistent Pain in Older Persons," *Journal of the American Geriatrics Society* 50(6), June 2002 supplement, pp. S205-S224.

American Pain Society (APS) "Guideline for the Management of Pain in Osteoarthritis, Rheumatoid Arthritis and Juvenile Chronic Arthritis, 2002." Available at www.ampainsoc.org/whatsnew/031502.htm

American Psychiatric Association (2004) "APA Responds to FDA's New Warning on Antidepressants," Press release, October 15, 2004, available at www.psych.org/news_room/press_releases/04-55apaonfdablackboxwarning.pdf [accessed May 3, 2005].

Bates, David W. (1998) "Editorial: Drugs and Adverse Reactions: How worried should we be?" *Journal of the American Medical Association*, v. 279, n. 15, p. 1216-1217.

Bombardier, Claire, et al. (2000) "Comparison of Upper Gastrointestinal Toxicity of Rofecoxib and Naproxen in Patients with Rheumatoid Arthritis." *The New England Journal of Medicine*, v. 343, n. 21, November 23, 2000.

Bresalier, Robert S. et al. (2005) "Cardiovascular Events Associated with Rofecoxib in a Colorectal Adenoma Chemoprevention Trial," *New England Journal of Medicine* 352, March 17, 2005, pp. 1092-1102.

Calfee, John E. and Ximena Pinell (2005) "The Significance of the Vioxx Withdrawal." American Enterprise Institute, Washington, D.C.

Chau, Ian, and David Cunningham (2002) "Cyclooxygenase Inhibition in Cancer: A Blind Alley or a New Therapeutic Reality?" *New England Journal of Medicine*, v. 346, n. 14, p. 1085-1087 (April 4).

Dalen, James E. (2002) "Selective Cox-2 Inhibitors, NSAIDs, Aspirin, and Myocardial Infarction," *Archives of Internal Medicine* 162(10), May 27, 2002, pp. 1091-1092.

Emery, P., C.J. Hawkey, and Andres Moore (2001) "Letter: Prescribing in the U.K.," *Lancet*, v. 357, p. 809 (March 10).

FitzGerald, Garret A. and Carlo Patrono. "The Coxibs, Selective Inhibitors of Cyclooxygenase-2." *New England Journal of Medicine* 345(6), August 9, 2001, pp. 433-442.

Food and Drug Administration, "Fact Sheet: FDA Improvements in Drug Safety Monitoring," February 15, 2005.

Food and Drug Administration, Press release, "Reforms Will Improve Oversight and Openness at FDA," February 15, 2005.

Food and Drug Administration, "FDA News: FDA Issues Final Risk Minimization Guidances." March 24, 2005, available at www.fda.gov/bbs/topics/news/2005/NEW01169.html

Food and Drug Administration, "Guidance for Industry: Development and Use of Risk Minimization Action Plans." March 2005, available at www.fda.gov/cder/guidance/6358fnl.htm

Food and Drug Administration, "Guidance for Industry: Good Pharmacovigilance Practices and Pharmacoepidemiologic Assessment." March 2005, available at www.fda.gov/cder/guidance/6359OCC.htm

Food and Drug Administration, "Guidance for Industry: Premarketing Risk Assessment." March 2005, available at www.fda.gov/cder/guidance/6357fnl.htm

Food and Drug Administration, "FDA Announces Series of Changes to the Class of Marketed Non-Steroidal Anti-Inflammatory Drugs (NSAIDs)," Press release, April 7, 2005, available at www.fda.gov/bbs/topics/news/2005/NEW01171.html. Accessed May 2, 2005.

Gurwitz, Jerry H., Terry S. Field, Leslie R. Harrold, Jeffrey Rothschild, Kristin Debellis, Andrew C. Seger, Cynthia Cadoret, Leslie S. Fish, Lawrence Garber, Michael Kelleher, and David W. Bates (2003) "Incidence and Preventability of Adverse Drug Events Among Older Persons in the Ambulatory Setting," *Journal of the American Medical Association*, v. 289, n. 9, p.1107-1116 (Mar. 5).

Jenkins, John K., and Paul J. Seligman (2005) "Analysis and Recommendations for Agency Action Regarding Non-steroidal Anti-inflammatory Drugs and Cardiovascular Risk," Food and Drug Administration, Center for Drug Evaluation and Research, Office of New Drugs, April 6, 2005.

Juni, Peter, Linda Nartey, Stephan Reichenbach, Rebekka Sterchi, Paul A. Dieppe, and Matthias Egger (2004) "Risk of Cardiovascular Events and Rofecoxib: Cumulative Meta-Analysis," *The Lancet*, v. 364, p. 2021-2029 (November 5, 2004).

Lancet, Dec. 4, 2004, "Editorial: Vioxx, the Implosion of Merck, and aftershocks at the FDA," v. 364, p. 1995-1996.

Lancet, Feb. 26, 2005, "Editorial: Safety Concerns at the FDA," v. 365, p. 727-728.

Leape, Lucian L. (2002) "Reporting of Adverse Events," *Journal of the American Medical Association*, v. 347, n. 20, p. 1633-1638 (November 14, 2002).

Leape, Lucian L. (2002) "Reporting of Adverse Events," *Journal of the American Medical Association*, v. 347, n. 20, p. 1633-1638 (November 14, 2002).

McClellan, Mark (2003) "FDA: Protecting and Advancing America's Health," Schroeder Lecture, October 7th, 2003, available at http:lawwww.cwru.edu/student_life/journals/health_matrix/142/McClellan.pdf [accessed May 3, 2005].

Merck, press release, "Merck Announces Voluntary Worldwide Withdrawal of VIOXX®" September 30, 2004.

Mukherjee, Debabrata, Steven E. Nissen, and Eric J. Topol. "Risk of Cardiovascular Events Associated with Selective Cox-2 Inhibitors." *Journal of the American Medical Association* 286(8), August 22, 2001, pp. 954-59.

New York Times, September 16, 2004, "Doctors Say They Will Cut Antidepressant Use," by Gardiner Harris.

New York Times, October 19, 2004. "A New Trial of Celebrex, and Questions on Its Timing," by Andrew Pollack.

New York Times, December 21, 2004, "Madison Ave. Sharing Drug Makers' Pain," by Nat Ives.

Pelayo, Juan Carlos. Memo to Sandra Cook et al. on "Consultation NDA 21-042 [Vioxx]" FDA Center for Drug Evaluation and Research, April 30, 1999.

Schnitzer, Thomas J. (2002) "Update of ACR Guidelines for Osteoarthritis: Role of the Coxibs," *Journal of Pain and Symptom Management*, v. 23, n. 4 (Supp. 1), p. S24-S30 (April 2002).

Scott, David G., and Riachard A. Watts (2005) "Letter: Increased Risk of Cardiovascular Events with Coxibs and NSAIDs," *Lancet*, v. 365, p. 1537 (April 30).

Topol, Eric J. (2004b) "Failing the Public Health: Rofecoxib, Merck, and the FDA," *New England Journal of Medicine*, v. 351, n. 17, p. 1707-1709 (October 21, 2004).

Wall Street Journal, April 12, 2005, "Dementia Drugs Get Warning," by Anna Wilde Mathews and Heather Won Tesoriero. [Black box warnings on seven anti-psychotic drugs used to treat dementia patients.]

Whittle, J.R. (2000) "COX-1 and COX-2 products in the gut; therapeutic impact of COX-2 inhibitors," *Gut*, v. 47, p. 320-325 (September).

Wolfe, M. Michael, David Lichtenstein, and Gurkirpal Singh (1999) "Gastrointestinal Toxicity of Nonsteriodal Anti-inflammatory Drugs," 340/24 *New England Journal of Medicine* 1888-1899.

Chairman TOM DAVIS. Dr. Calfee, thank you very much.
Dr. Wilkes.

STATEMENT OF MICHAEL WILKES, M.D., PH.D.

Dr. WILKES. Thank you, Mr. Chairman and members of the committee. It is a pleasure to be here, and I hope I can provide you with some insight from my perspective. I come to you as a dean overseeing medical education of doctors at all levels, as a medical school teacher, a practicing doctor of internal medicine, and a former medical journal editor.

Pharmaceutical expenditures are the fastest growing part of healthcare, about 15 percent a year. About 8 percent of healthcare costs are spent on drugs, much of this coming out of consumers' pockets. A conservative estimate is that Pharma spent $20 billion on drug marketing and promotion, or, as Pharma prefers to call it, "educational outreach." During this same time, all the U.S. medical schools combined spent only $3.5 billion educating doctors. If you add in residencies, we spent $3.9 billion, still half of what Pharma spent on education.

How do doctors learn about new drugs? Well, once a doctor completes their training, there really is no formal system, it is all independent, it is "catch as catch can"; and this is where Pharma steps in. But after all is said and done, what we really need to focus on isn't corporate profits or what doctors are prescribing, it is people's health.

For doctors who write a prescription when no drug is needed, or who choose a drug when the patient can't afford the drug, or who use a newer drug when an older one is better or more effective, the end result is the same: poor quality care. There is example after example where, despite sound guiding evidence, doctors write prescriptions for bad drugs: beta blockers, finasteride, diabetes drugs, fluoroquinolones, calcium channel blockers, dementia drugs like Aricept, TPA, and the wrong indications.

How does all of this happen? Well, lots of explanations. First let us look at doctors and drug reps, and how they interact. In chemistry class, when we study a chemical reaction that has many different steps, the step that limits the speed of the reaction, the most important step, is called the "rate-limiting step."

In medicine, the rate-limiting step for pharmaceutical corporate profits is the doctor; it is he or she, after all, who writes the prescription. If companies can't change their behavior, profits suffer. Pharma, as we have heard, has an army 88,000 strong who are on the front lines with doctors trying to convince them to write prescriptions for their product. That is one rep for every six doctors, or $9,000 per every doctor in this country.

Now, why should drug promotion be different than, say, car promotion? When a bright person decides to buy a car, they shop around; they might read Consumer's Reports, they might talk to the car salesman. The consumer decides what engine they want; they decide what color they want; what model they want. Short of being fraudulent or lying, everybody knows the car salesman is there to sell cars; the buyer must beware. But no one expects a car salesman to act in the public's best interest; they are there to sell cars.

As a profession, medicine is profoundly different. We have a covenant with society to act in their best interest. We go to school for years and years, and we are expected to use our knowledge to benefit the public. We interpret and explain the risks and benefits of treatments so that a sick person can decide for themselves what action they wish to take. The doctor is supposed to be in the patient's corner. But when we let our own self interest get in the way, we break that covenant with society and we invite public outrage and oversight. All of the gifts—the trips, the tickets, the lunches—all contribute to breaking the doctor's trust with the public.

Now, the information that we are provided, is it accurate? One has to first decide how one defines accurate. If we are going to hold drug ads to the same level as Volvos, Coke, or Crest toothpaste, then perhaps we are OK. But if we are going to hold Pharma to the standard of being educational, then their ads need to be held to the same high standards of educational material in medicine: it needs to be peer-reviewed, it needs to be highly factually accurate, and it needs to be clear.

Medical education and CME—continuing medical education—is required in nearly all States in this country. That is because new knowledge becomes outdated very quickly. While CME has become an important part of doctors' professional lives, Pharma money has become the lifeline of CME. In all of this, Pharma maintains it is providing an educational service. But is it an educational service if Pharma provides the food, chooses the speakers, trains the speakers, provides the slides for the speakers to use, sets the agenda, and if they prohibit debate and don't allow alternative explanations?

Does promotion have an effect on drug sales? I guess the obvious question is of course it does. Why else would Pharma spend $20 billion? Some studies have tried to answer this by observing prescribing changes before, during and after promotional activities. These are relatively simple studies, they are inexpensive, and they provide convincing evidence that promotion works. A researcher named Cleary looked at what happens to prescribing before and after drug salesmen come and go. He found a profound effect.

Of course, the ideal way to find out about the impact of promotion on prescribing is to ask the manufacturers to experimentally do promotional activities in one part of the country and then compare that with other regions. And there is no doubt that Pharma has done this; the problem is the information is proprietary and we don't have access to it. Nonetheless, it seems clear to everyone that promotion leads to increased sales.

In conclusion, pharmaceutical promotion provides neither education, nor does it enhance the quality of medical care. In fact, as we have heard today, there is evidence that drug promotion may actually deter high-quality care. Professional organizations of doctors and medical journals in academic medicine have been bought out by the generous gifts and bribes offered by Pharma. Doctors have accepted promotions in lieu of bona fide education because it suits our desires not our needs, and it feeds doctors' egos. The conflicts of interest are significant, they are real, and they are obvious. Relying on drug companies for unbiased evaluations about their product makes no more sense to me than relying on Vodka manufacturers to each us about alcoholism.

We know that government regulation of promotion is far more effective than industry self-regulation, but it only works when the government has teeth and isn't afraid to use them. Medical education, hospitals, government, medical journals, and the great medical societies of our country all are partially to blame for the mess that we are in with regard to educating doctors about drugs, and they all have to be part of the solution.

It is difficult for me to think of any other area in commerce where false and misleading advertising and promotion can do as much damage as it can with pharmaceutical promotions.

Thank you.

[The prepared statement of Dr. Wilkes follows:]

Testimony of Michael Wilkes, M.D., Ph.D.
Vice Dean, Medical Education
Professor of Medicine and Public Health
May 4th 2005

Chairman Davis and Members of the Committee on Government Reform, I thank you for the opportunity to testify today. I have been asked to address issues related to the impact of pharmaceutical promotions on physician prescribing and the quality and cost of health care from my perspective as a medical school dean, an educator, a medical researcher, and a former medical journal editor.

Pharmaceutical expenditures are the fastest growing part of health care costs increasing at 15% a year. Americans spend 8% their health care dollars on drugs – much of this coming out of their own pockets. A conservative estimate is that last year Pharma spent $20 billion dollars on drug marketing and promotion or as Pharma prefers to call it "educational outreach". During this same time period all the US medical schools spent only $3.5 on medical education and residencies spent $3.9 billion on education (calculations based on demographic data provided in personal communication AAMC). This $20 billion is far more than is spent on research and development, and is more than is spent on manufacturing and distribution. Promotional (marketing) money is divided between promoting drug products to physicians and promoting the same products to the public. Most of the following presentation will focus on physician-Pharma interactions but DTC advertising is not to be overlooked as an enormous source of misleading information that results in inappropriate medical care with a huge impact on medical costs, patient expectations, and iatrogenic illness.

How do doctors learn about new drugs?

In an ideal world medical schools would teach students to make prescribing decisions based on the best available evidence taking in to account benefits, risks, costs, and mechanisms of action. In fact, medical schools spend shockingly little time teaching doctors in training about rational prescribing. In four years of medical school, less than 5% of actual teaching time relates to the use of medications. Once a doctor completes her training there is no formal, independent system to teach doctors about new drugs and treatments. It is catch as catch can. This is where Pharma has stepped in. Not surprisingly, the prescribing practices of most physicians and physicians in training are heavily influenced by $20 billion spent on drug promotion.

The end result of Pharma's major role in educating doctors about prescription drugs is poor, dangerous, and overly expensive prescribing practices of American physicians. There are example after example of where, despite sound evidence, doctors write prescriptions for inferior but heavily marketed products (beta blockers, finasteride, diabetes drugs, fluoroquinolones, calcium channel blocking drugs, dementia drugs, TPA, etc.) ignoring or being unaware of the scientific evidence.

How effective are physician – drug rep interactions

In chemistry class when we study chemical reactions the step, in a multistep reaction, that limits the speed of the reaction is called the "rate-limiting step". In medicine, the rate-limiting step leading to increased drugs sales is the doctor who, after all, writes the prescription. Pharma currently employs an army of 88,000 sales reps who are on the front lines with doctors convincing them to write prescriptions for expensive drugs, occasionally dangerous drugs, and often drugs that are far less effective than alternatives. There is one drug rep for every six physicians or thought of in economic terms Pharma spends about $9000 per doctor per year. Perhaps more appropriate for Congressional consideration is whether prescription drug costs would be substantially lower if we did away with this costly promotion. Lower drug costs would almost certainly translate in to more people getting the drugs they really need.

Drug reps (detailers) are usually gregarious, young, and attractive. And they are well schooled in persuasion. Written manuals, videos, and simulation exercises are just a few of the trench warfare tools used to teach detailers how to engage doctors in the field. Detailers are usually found roaming hospital hallways or paying visits to doctors' offices. Dressed in their conservative business attire they almost always come with gifts including free samples, flowers for the front office staff (who are crucial in helping to arrange for the doctor to meet the rep), lunches, books, loads of pens, and invitations to dinners, sporting events and trips. There are even examples of drug companies actually paying doctors to prescribe their drug.

As a child, my mother told me I couldn't buy anything advertised on TV. She explained that if the product was really that good the manufacturer wouldn't need to spend all that money telling everyone how good it was. The same is true for drugs. Very few drugs being advertised are any great shakes. In fact, most medical professors tell our students to avoid prescribing any new drugs until its use can be tested and established in the real world of medical practice as opposed to pharmaceutically sponsored drug studies. Advertising is meant to sell drugs and the less effective the drug the more marketing it takes to sell it.

Why should drug promotion be different from car promotion?

When a bright person decides to purchase a car they shop around, they read Consumer's Report, and they talk to the car salesmen. The consumer decides what size engine, what color, and what model they want. Short of lying or being fraudulent the car salesmen is there to sell cars and the buyer must beware. No one expects a car salesman to act in the public's interest – they are only there to sell cars.

As a profession, medicine is profoundly different. We have a covenant with society to act in society's best interest. Doctors go to school for years to learn their science. And we use that science for the public's benefit. We interpret and explain the risks and benefits of a treatment so that a sick person can decide what course of action they wish to take. The patient needs the doctor solidly in their corner.

In exchange for all this hard work and for acting selflessly, doctors are given lots of privileges. Doctors are paid handsomely, they have all the rights of a profession including deciding who gets in to the profession and who can call themselves doctors.

But once we let our own self-interest get in the way we break our covenant with society and we invite public outrage and oversight. All these gifts, trips, tickets, and lunches have compromised the public's trust.

How accurate is the information provided by Pharma to doctors?

First, one has to decide what standard should be applied to promotional information. If they are "just ads", then perhaps they should be held to no higher standard than the promotional material for Volvos, Coke, or Crest toothpaste. If, as is maintained by Pharma, their material is "educational" then their ads need to be held to the high standards of educational material that usually includes peer review, high factual accuracy, and clarity.

In fact, promotional material is not meeting these standards. As Former FDA Commissioner Kessler described, "…enormous potential exists for misleading advertisements to reach the physician and influence prescribing decisions…misleading advertisements can result in significant adverse consequences…needless injury or even death may occur because physicians have been persuaded to prescribe products for uses for which they have not been adequately tested or to substitute therapies that may be less safe or less effective than the alternatives.

Stryer and Bero showed that much information (42%) failed to comply with one or more FDA regulation including 35%, which lacked fair balance between risks and benefits. My research has shown that 40% of print ads in medical journals did not present fair balance, 58% contained images that expert reviewers felt minimized concerns about side effects, and that 47% of the ads did not appropriately highlight risks and contraindications in special populations such as the elderly. Few ads addressed cost. Collectively, these research findings are typical of this body of literature.

What impact does pharmaceutical promotion have on doctors' knowledge?

Studies, including several that I have conducted, show that lots of promotional material contains inaccuracies, or at least presents very selective accounts of the evidence about the drug. Do these inaccuracies impact on patient's health?

Traditionally doctors report using three sources of information to find out about new drugs -- materials from sales representatives, CME conferences, and journal advertisements. How these sources are used depends upon the specialty of the physician and on the age of the doctor. Those in practice more than 15 years tend to rely more heavily on drug sales representatives as a source of information about new drugs while more recent grads tend to rely on CME courses. Several reports suggest that drug promotional material is often used as a primary source of information for new drugs, especially for conditions for which the doctor is uncertain. These are precisely the conditions when we would want our doctor reading a reliable source or talking with an expert (pharmacist).

Doesn't it make sense for doctors to learn directly from the pharmaceutical industry?

There is no question that doctors are inadequately trained to use medications. Most medical schools under teach clinical pharmacology, and more importantly, few of us teach medical students or residents how to appropriately use the expertise of pharmacists.

From a pharmaceutical manufacturer's perspective *education* is about teaching the "clinically naive" how to start using your outstandingly beneficial product. Such activities are not educational in the slightest. They are pure promotion and in fact the funds for this "education" come from the companies' *marketing budgets*. This is contrary to how medical schools teach our trainees. The mantra in medical education is "evidence based curriculum" – in other words teach what the independent, non biased studies actually show about a drugs effectiveness when compared to the most commonly used alternative drugs. Medical educators are working to revise and update our teaching.

But educating the huge number of practicing physicians is far more difficult. Continuing Medical Education (CME) is a requirement for doctors in nearly all states. This is because medicine is not a fixed science but an evolving art. New knowledge quickly supplants old and doctors, who would otherwise choose to see more patients, are often hesitant to take time off to study and learn new material. CME has become an important part of doctors' professional lives and Pharma money has become the life-line of CME. As every editor of a medical journal knows, and most providers of CME know, doctors are hesitant – some might say unwilling – to pay a fee for quality learning material. This is why journals are dependent upon advertising revenue and why professional societies such as the AMA, the American College of Physicians, Society for Critical Care Medicine and the Thyroid Society are all beholden to drug companies. The recent prestigious American College of Physicians (ACP) annual meeting had nearly every event and every possible minute underwritten by Pharma. In fact, in contrast to their written ethical standards they chose to promote themselves to drug companies with the following claim, "…an unparalleled opportunity to meet physicians with power…prescribing power".

The medical profession and Pharma have an unhealthy symbiotic relationship that is pulling down the medical profession. The professional groups provide the doctors and the drug companies provide the money. Medical journals, medical societies, and even medical schools fight to woo drug company sponsorship of educational events. Without their sponsorship CME activities would be more basic, less high-tech, and perhaps it would cost a bit more to attend but they would be honest, accurate, and trustworthy.

Pharma maintains it is providing an "educational service" – even though Pharma provides the food, the speakers, the slides, and the agenda. But it takes two to tango and the medical profession – particularly academic medicine should be embarrassed. We've allowed our faculty to become tainted – rather than insisting they be the arbiters of goodness and truth. We've allowed our training mission to serve a dual mission – true education and Pharma promotion.

Why do doctors interact with pharmaceutical reps?

There are three reasons: 1) free food and perks, 2) doctors feel they deserve such gifts, and 3) reps often fill a perceived educational need.

The power of free food is not to be overlooked. Doctors and trainees work long hours and often skip lunch. In community hospitals, academic medical centers, Veterans Hospitals and clinics drug reps bring free food. They also hand out promotional material and shmooze with the doctors. Sometimes the drug reps give a 15-minute presentation. Companies often invite doctors to lavish restaurants to hear these presentations. Merck held such events often to promote their cox-2 inhibitor Vioxx and when asked about the cardiovascular dangers of the drug they downplayed any harm.

Doctors often perceive that they "deserve" these benefits since they are, after all, working long hard hours on behalf of their patients. Little thought is given to the huge cost that patients incur in paying for these meals and gifts that of course are part of the patients' high drug prices.

A recent study in the Annals of Internal Medicine (Feb 2005) explains why older physicians are less likely to deliver high-quality care. Medical advances occur frequently, and the explicit knowledge that physicians possess may easily become out of date. Therefore, although it is generally assumed that the tacit knowledge and skills accumulated by physicians during years of practice lead to superior clinical abilities, it has been shown that physicians with more experience may paradoxically be less likely to provide technically appropriate care. This applies most particularly to prescribing drugs. Doctors are aware that they quickly become out of date and seek easy ways to keep up to date. Pharma seeks to provide "a feel good" approach to learning about new medicines. Unfortunately, the information they provide is insufficient to educate a doctor. Comparisons between new and existing drugs are rare, and information is spun so as to make newer drugs sound far superior and safe. In fact, only a very small percentage of new drugs offer any substantial benefit over existing drugs.

Why are doctors willing to accept information from pharmaceutical reps?

My research has shown that the courtship between Pharma and doctors in training starts early in medical school. Medical students are poor, overworked, and want to feel important. Drug companies sponsor mixers and "liver rounds" (aka parties), provides free pens, books, and medical equipment and even free prescription drugs all intended to appeal to the desires of medical students (relaxation, entitlement, and kindness). All of this is provided early and often through the medical school years without any expectation of directly impacting on prescribing; after all students are several steps removed from the actual writing of prescriptions – at least for the time being. However, the goal is to curry favor and prepare a futile soil for the future. Sandberg found that students given textbooks by pharmaceutical sales representatives are unlikely to remember the name of the company or its products. However, the gift establishes habits, e.g. a willingness to receive gifts and the development of positive attitudes towards drug companies. This is the medical equivalent of feeding the bears in the National Parks. After just a few time of compassionate feeding the bears learn to keep coming back. In fact, they forget how to find food on their own. Doctors have become the health care system's educational "bears".

Once students graduate and they can prescribe drugs research shows promotional material is highly effective at altering prescribing patterns. Yet despite a large amount of research that documents a profound effect of promotion on doctor's prescribing habits doctors commonly deny that their prescribing decisions are in any way influenced by promotional material. Why? Because they want the lunches and they feel entitled.

What role has organized medicine and academic medicine taken to limit physician – Pharma interactions?

In recent years the pharmaceutical industry's marketing tactics have come to the public's attention. Books by Angell, Kassirer, Avorn, and others have received national attention. Conflicts of interest at the NIH and other academic institutions have made national headlines. In response some organizations including the AMA and the ACP have introduced new guidelines to limit real and perceived conflicts of interest. In 2002 the Pharmaceutical Manufacturers Association reissued its own strengthened guidelines to cut back on bribery. But for the most part all these guidelines are window dressing intended to get the public and policy makers off their backs. Because these organizations have come to depend on industry money for their life blood there is little chance of meaningful change without strict new policies and federal oversight. Recall the example mention above involving the 2005 annual ACP meeting and its relationship with Pharma. On the one hand the organization issues strict rules about doctors relations with drug companies but on the other hand it promotes and court that same money. The same conflicts of interest exist at JAMA, the NEJM, UCLA, NYY, Harvard and nearly every other American medical school.

Does pharmaceutical promotion impact on doctor's prescribing behaviors?

This is a difficult area to research but the answer is an unequivocal "yes". The outcome that is most important to measure is does the doctor write a prescription for a new product -- not whether or not she can answer some multiple choice questions. Most doctors are unaware of how much promotion they are exposed to. Surveys based on self-report are appropriate for finding out what people think is happening, or how they want to present themselves, but not what really happens in doctors offices or hospitals.

The outcomes that matter in terms of measuring promotion's effectiveness include 1) impact of promotion on the doctor's prescribing behavior, 2) impact of promotion on overall drug sales, and 3) physician's requests for additions to the pharmacy formulary.

A useful group of studies look at specific drugs and how they are promoted. From an industry perspective, a successful promotion results in positive changes in individual prescribing behavior. Bower and Burkett found that family physicians who reported relying less on drug sales representatives for information were likely to prescribe more generic drugs, as were residency trained doctors, and regular readers of weekly medical journals. Those who engaged in more appropriate and rational prescribing held more positive attitudes toward generics, and gave other indications of a less positive attitude towards the industry and promotion, than other doctors. Researcher found that the answer to a single question (are sales representatives a good sources of prescribing information about new drugs?) was most predictive of appropriate prescribing.

In summary, there is strong evidence that doctors who rely on promotion as a source of information about drugs, prescribe more drugs, prescribe less rationally, and prescribe new drugs earlier than other doctors. Two researchers (Orlowski and Wateska) looked at the impact of educational symposia on physician prescribing and their report is described this way:

> *Using the hospital pharmacy inventory, they tracked the use of two drugs within one institution 22 months before and 17 months after each symposium about them. They also collected data on the national usage of these drugs, and informally interviewed the doctors who had gone to the symposia. Most of the doctors said that the symposia would not influence their prescribing, but some said that they might make them think of the drug more and the symposium might convince them of the benefits of the drug. Orlowski and Wateska found a dramatic and statistically highly significant increase in the use of the drugs in the hospital after the relevant symposia. These increases were not reflected in national data, and they did not seem to affect the hospital's use of alternative drugs. This study provides evidence firstly, that exposure to promotion increases prescribing, and secondly that it can do so whether or not those exposed consider themselves vulnerable to such influence.*

Does promotion have an impact on overall drug sales?

Perhaps the most obvious answer to this question is "well, of course it does, why else would drug companies spend $20 billion dollars!"

Some studies have tried to answer this question by observing prescribing changes before, during or after promotional activities. These studies are relatively simple and inexpensive and provide convincing evidence of the impact on promotion. Cleary looked at what happened when the level of promotion varied naturally over time, say when a sales representative was away on a sales training course. He examined trends in numbers of new prescriptions for three third-generation antibiotics in one hospital. He found that when the sales representative was away the numbers of new prescriptions for this product dropped. This did not happen to the other products studied, and there was no correlation between the pattern in this hospital or regional or national sales. Dieperink and

Drogemuller looked at one psychiatric medicine. They found that the reason for a dramatic increase in the use of an atypical antipsychotic agent in their Minneapolis hospital was a Grand Rounds presentation sponsored by the manufacturer of the product.

Of course the ideal way to find out about the impact of promotion on prescribing is to ask manufacturers to experimentally vary promotion over regions and times, monitor the effect of this and publish the results. There is no doubt that drug companies have done this many times over, but the information is proprietary. None-the-less, it seems clear that promotion leads to increased sales.

Are promotions aimed at doctors the only effective way to alter drug prescribing?

No. Direct to consumer advertising (DTCA) is the fastest growing part of the advertising pie accounting for 20% ($8 billion) of promotional activities (depending on how you count other activities). Like other promotional activities, the vast majority of advertised products are for new, expensive, "me-to" drugs that have little if any benefit over older more reliable drugs. The evidence that DTAs work is overwhelming. It works at defining disease, it works at setting patient expectations that they need a drug for their disease, it works at guilting doctors in to writing a prescription so as to maintain patient satisfaction or saving time, and most importantly, it works at selling drugs.

A growing number of studies have examined the effects of DTC advertising on consumer and clinician behavior, but few have directly addressed the issue of overprescribing. Last week we published in JAMA a randomized controlled trial using standardized patients (SPs) to address 3 research questions:
     (1) What are the effects of patients' requests for a prescription on physician prescribing?
     (2) Does it make a difference whether patients' requests are brand-specific (as might be prompted by viewing a DTC television advertisement) or general (as might arise from watching a television program about a health condition)?
     (3) What are the effects of brand-specific and general requests on 2 other health care indicators: referral and follow-up?

The results confirm that patients' requests have a profound effect on physician prescribing, quality of medical care, and health care costs.

A major problem with DTCA is that there is no one at home guarding the hen's and the fox is running around wild in the hen house. The FDA does not take their responsibility to monitor these medical messages seriously. It has less than 40 experts to review tens of thousands of print and electronic promotions. Even when the FDA does send out a disciplinary letter it is rarely effective at changing the manufacturers' behavior. My research has shown that the public strongly believes that the FDA is monitoring and correcting drug advertisements to assure their accuracy in ways not done with other products.

CONCLUSION

In conclusion, pharmaceutical promotions provide neither education nor enhance the quality of medical care – and there is evidence drugs ads may actually deter high quality care. Professional organizations of doctors, medical journals, and academic medicine have been bought out by the generous gifts provided by Pharma. Doctors have accepted drug "promotions" in lieu of bona fide education because it suits our desires (but not our needs) and it feeds our egos. The conflicts of interest are significant and obvious. Relying on drug companies for unbiased evaluations of their products makes no more sense than relying on vodka manufacturers to teach us about alcoholism. Pharma does not function in a free market and the playing field is not even. As such the government needs to assure a more equitable balance between the interests of shareholders and those of the public.

Doctors need to perceive that small gifts from drug company reps are not acceptable and profoundly influence prescribing choices. Few patients think *THEIR* doctor receives these promotional gifts; if they discovered this they report they would hold their doctor in lower regard. Perhaps this offers an opportunity to educate the public with the hope of altering physician behavior.

We know that government regulation of promotion is far more effective than industry self-regulation but only when the government (FDA) has teeth and isn't afraid to use them. Journals can, but won't, subject promotional material to the same sort of rigorous peer review as other educational material. Such a move risks offending advertisers and no journal has taken this responsible step -- all continue to publish misleading promotional information and claim it is not their responsibility to address accuracy or bias. In fact, journals actively promote themselves to Pharma as the most effective way to change doctor's prescribing habits. Perhaps this is another good reason to require that all federally funded research be placed on PubMed Central with free public access and no commercial sponsorship.

It is difficult to think of any other area of commerce where false and misleading advertising and promotion can do as much damage as it can with pharmaceutical promotions.

References:

1. Bower AD, Burkett GL. Family physicians and generic drugs: a study of recognition, information sources, prescribing attitudes, and practices. J Fam Pract 1987;24:612-6.
2. Berings D, Blondeel L, Habraken H. The effect of industry-independent drug information on the prescribing of benzodiazepines in general practice. Eur J Clin Pharmacol 1994;46:501-505.
3. Caamano, F.; Figueiras, A., and Gestal-Otero, J. J. Influence of commercial information on prescription quantity in primary care. Eur J Public Health. 2002 Sep; 12(3):187-91.
4. Watkins, C. Harvey, I. Carthy, P. Moore, L. Robinson, E. Brawn, R. Attitudes and behaviour of general practitioners and their prescribing costs a national cross sectional survey. Qual Saf Health Care. 2003 Feb; 12(1)29-34.
5. Lipton S, Boyd EA, Bero LA. Conflicts of interest in academic research: policies, processes, and attitudes. Account Res. 2004 Apr-Jun;11(2):83-102.

6. Lexchin J, Bero LA, Djulbegovic B, Clark O. Pharmaceutical industry sponsorship and research outcome and quality: systematic review. BMJ. 2003 May 31;326(7400):1167-70. Review.

7. Rochon PA, Bero LA, Bay AM, Gold JL, Dergal JM, Binns MA, Streiner DL, Gurwitz JH. Comparison of review articles published in peer-reviewed and throwaway journals. JAMA. 2002 Jun 5;287(21):2853-6.

8. Bero LA. "Educational" advertisements--I haven't seen one yet! West J Med. 2001 Jun;174(6):395.

9. Boyd EA, Bero LA. Assessing faculty financial relationships with industry: A case study. JAMA. 2000 Nov 1;284(17):2209-14.

10. Stryer D, Bero LA. Characteristics of materials distributed by drug companies. An evaluation of appropriateness. J Gen Intern Med. 1996 Oct;11(10):575-83.

11. Wilkes, M.S., Bell, R., and Kravitz, R. "Direct to Consumer Advertising: Trends, Impact, and

12. Implications" Health Affairs Journal March 2000;19:110-128

13. Bell, R.A., Kravitz, R.L., Wilkes, M.S. "Direct-to-Consumer prescription drug advertising, 1989-1998. A Content Analysis of Conditions, Targets, Inducements, and Appeals" Journal of Family Practice 2000;49(4):329-35

14. Wilkes MS, Hoffman JR. An innovative approach to educating medical students about pharmaceutical promotion. Acad Med. 2001 Dec;76(12):1271-7.

Chairman TOM DAVIS. Well, thank you, too, very much, Dr. Wilkes. A lot of interesting perspectives on the panel.

Dr. Erb, I am going to start with you, and I will set it for 10 minutes. I am going to ask you to turn to exhibit Tab 9. Refer to it. After VIGOR, Merck prepared bulletins for its sales force. In those—and if you turn to Tab 9 as one example—in the first paragraph you tell your sales force not to initiate discussions on the FDA's Arthritis Advisory Committee or the results of the VIGOR study.

Now, in another bulletin under Tab 4, which has the CV card behind the bulletin—and the CV card is also on Tab 5—Merck instructs its sales force to utilize the cardiovascular card [CV], when answering physicians' questions regarding the CV risk for Vioxx.

This card does not contain data from VIGOR, is that correct?

Mr. ERB. That is correct. The data in that card is the data that was from studies that formed the basis of the approval of the NDA and the approved label at that point in time.

Chairman TOM DAVIS. So was Merck doing anything to inform physicians about the results of VIGOR?

Mr. ERB. Yes. We fully disclosed the results for VIGOR. Within 2 weeks after knowing the results, we issued a press release that described both the GI benefits and also the cardiovascular——

Chairman TOM DAVIS. In fact, this was widely written up in a lot of different papers, wasn't it, in medical journals?

Mr. ERB. That is correct. We also presented it in a number of scientific forms and wrote up a paper which was published that year in the New England Journal of Medicine. So it did get very wide distribution.

Chairman TOM DAVIS. And a wide awake physician would have obviously known about this, wouldn't they?

Mr. ERB. That is correct, yes.

Chairman TOM DAVIS. How did the CV card assist this? A CV card didn't assist, though, in giving them information, did it?

Mr. ERB. Well, the CV card—let me start with in our commitment to promote within accordance to our label and the laws and regulations, we promote information that is in the approved application and approved label. The CV card, the data in that CV card was the information from the original trials that supported the Vioxx approval, as well as the current label at that point in time.

The VIGOR trial was a trial that we developed in order to show the GI benefits, and it also studied the safety of the compound.

Chairman TOM DAVIS. VIGOR was 1 of 70 trials, is that right?

Mr. ERB. VIGOR was 1 of 70 trials. The VIGOR trial was specifically initiated to change the label to show that the benefits we saw in our endoscopy studies in the original submission translated into a clinical benefit too. We also showed in that study, too, the safety of the compound and the cardiovascular risks. Given our commitment to promote in accordance to the label, we gave specific instructions, since the label had not been approved yet with the VIGOR information in it, that our sales force should not have that discussion.

However, it was widely distributed, in scientific forums as well as press releases and in the New England Journal of Medicine, and if a physician asked an unsolicited question about VIGOR, we have tools, such as a professional information request, where the physician's questions can be answered with headquarters material, even though the sales representatives could not speak to them at that point in time.

Chairman TOM DAVIS. Did you have anything on your Web site? I mean, it seems to me a lot of physicians would have asked about VIGOR after reading this.

Mr. ERB. That is correct. And in the time since the VIGOR submission, we had approximately 123,000 requests for professional information requests. So these are physicians——

Chairman TOM DAVIS. You couldn't very well hide it at that point, even though it was not on the card.

Mr. ERB. No. This is why it was picked up in the press and it was very widely disclosed, yes.

Chairman TOM DAVIS. Who created the CV card? Do you know where that came from?

Mr. ERB. It comes from our marketing department, but it is also approved through our medical legal board, and our medical legal board consists of a lawyer and two physicians to make sure that the information in there is balanced, accurate, and is consistent with the approved label that we have at that point in time.

Chairman TOM DAVIS. Explain to me what Merck did after the VIGOR study to ensure the safety and the efficacy of Vioxx. This presented a kind of problem that I don't know if you anticipated, but obviously this is your study that you went ahead with to try to ascertain what the facts were. How did Merck—you made the results public right away.

Mr. ERB. For the VIGOR study are you talking about?

Chairman TOM DAVIS. Yes. Because I think that is what is central to the questions about how the FDA handled it and how you handled it.

Mr. ERB. Right. We base our scientific evaluation and scientific investigation on some basic principles, such as disclosure, which we have just talked about, as well as monitoring and studying the compound. Since the VIGOR findings, we actually did both animal studies as well as continued to assess the cardiovascular safety in our ongoing clinical studies at that point in time. We had clinical studies ongoing that included placebo as a control. Two of those studies were Alzheimer's disease study, which were also incorporated into the approved label when VIGOR data was incorporated into it. And we didn't see in those studies any difference in cardiovascular risk.

We also had several other large long-term studies ongoing versus placebo, too, that were going to form the basis of an analysis of the cardiovascular risks of the compound. So we extensively studied the product afterwards, and, as I mentioned before, we conducted over 70 studies on over 40,000 patients.

Chairman TOM DAVIS. How many patients were in the VIGOR study?

Mr. ERB. The VIGOR study included 8,000 patients. It was 4,000 both arms: 4,000 in the Vioxx arm, which was 50 milligrams, twice the recommended dose; and 4,000 in the naproxen arm, which was 500 milligrams twice a day.

Chairman TOM DAVIS. Can you explain what happened during the label negotiations and why they took so long to complete?

Mr. ERB. Well, I think how you have to look at that is to start from the beginning. We determined the results in March, and within 4 months submitted an application to the agency. The agency rigorously reviewed the application; they asked numerous questions and requests. We had approximately 50 requests for additional either analysis or clarifications, and many of those had multiple items on those, which we responded very rapidly to those.

There was also, during that timeframe, two studies that were ongoing, one study on Alzheimer's Disease patients and another one on mild cognitive impairment patients, which compared Vioxx versus placebo. And we felt that those studies—and so did the agency—were very relevant to the questions that were being asked. Since they were ongoing, we took interim analysis of those to provide to the agency, and we continued to update those in a safety update report and respond to the agency's questions on that.

When the agency reached a state where they felt they had the full information that they needed to enter into labeling discussions, we did so. And then we worked together in very good faith to provide that information in the label in a manner that is balanced, appropriate, and helpful for physicians.

Chairman TOM DAVIS. What was Merck's basis for promoting the theory of naproxen's potential cardiovascular protective effect in explaining the statistical difference between the CV events in naproxen and Vioxx in the VIGOR study?

Mr. ERB. Well, at that point in time, when we looked at the totality and the weight of the evidence that we had versus Vioxx versus placebo, Vioxx versus other NSAIDs other than naproxen, we did not see any difference in the cardiovascular risks. We do know that naproxen at the doses we were using, 500 milligrams twice a day, resulted in sustained blockage of anti-platelet aggregation, similar to what occurs in aspirin.

There was also other NSAIDs who show that same effect, which were shown to be cardio-protective. So we felt that the weight of the evidence at that point in time, since it was a controlled trial versus naproxen, that it was naproxen's cardio-protective benefit that was causing the differential there.

Chairman TOM DAVIS. OK. There has been a lot of discussion over the safety of Vioxx. Can you discuss the benefits of the drug and whether or not Merck plans to return Vioxx to the market?

Mr. ERB. Well, Vioxx is the only NSAID that has a clinically proven outcome in reducing the risk of serious gastrointestinal bleeds and ulcers. We feel that is a unique benefit for Vioxx, and we are in preliminary discussions with the agency at this point in time to see what information they would require for their consideration of putting Vioxx back onto the marketplace.

Chairman TOM DAVIS. Thank you very much.

Dr. Calfee, in your testimony you state that too many warnings on a drug label can lead to as much harm as too few warnings; it leads to the under-use or the under-prescribing of effective drugs. How does FDA reach an appropriate balance between caution and unnecessary concern?

Mr. CALFEE. With great difficulty. It is just a very, very difficult task. The FDA is very clear from a lot of their public statements, and also from their actions, that they worry a lot about the over-warning effect. They worry a lot about labels that are getting cluttered with lots of warnings; physicians can't take them all into account.

And I know that in connection with the SSRI suicidality warning that there is concern within the agency and outside the agency that the effect might well be to discourage people from taking antidepressants that would help them a great deal, and there is a lot of at least anecdotal evidence that kind of thing actually happens. So it is a very difficult task for them, and it is very easy for them to err on the wrong side.

Chairman TOM DAVIS. Thank you very much. I have more questions, but my time is up.

Mr. Waxman, you have 10 minutes.

Mr. WAXMAN. Thank you, Mr. Chairman.

We have heard on many occasions from the pharmaceutical manufacturers, research association, and drug companies themselves that it is essential to allow physicians to have information about new drugs so that they can prescribe them appropriately, and that is the mission of the sales reps; and that, I think, is what Merck's lawyers have been saying as well. Our mission is to educate doctors.

Now, I look at the documents that we have received and I get a different picture: the goal is sales, not education. I would like to have you turn to Document 9. This is a bullet that Merck sent out to all field personnel with responsibility for Vioxx. The date is February 9, 2001, the day after an FDA advisory panel met in part to discuss the cardiovascular risks of the drug. This committee recommended that physicians be informed about the results of the VIGOR study, which found a fivefold increase in heart attacks among patients on Vioxx compared to naproxen.

Yet, Merck instructs its sales force of thousands—3,000, as I understand it—do not initiate discussions on the FDA Arthritis Advisory Committee review or the results of the VIGOR study. So the sales force is being instructed not to tell the doctors about this new information.

Now if you would turn to the last page of this document. It says if doctors ask about the cardiovascular findings of the VIGOR study, if they ask about it, Merck instructs their representatives to state "I can't discuss this study with you."

Dr. Wilkes, you are the vice dean of the medical education at University of California-Davis. If the purpose of pharmaceutical marketing were to educate physicians, would it make sense to tell the representatives not to discuss these findings with the doctors?

Dr. WILKES. No, it would make no sense. I think that one needs to be insightful to understand that doctors in America are working very hard, and they are looking for shortcuts and looking for quick answers, and that is when the pharmaceutical manufacturers have found a niche. They are looking to give doctors quick answers, doctors who really don't have the insight to understand the science, and if they truly are interested in educating them, they would be providing them with balanced evidence-based approach.

Mr. WAXMAN. Well, wait a second. Merck put out a press release; they had a forum on this subject, they sponsored a scientific forum; they had a paper published in the New England Journal of Medicine. These are widely available documents. Why wouldn't doctors just get that information from those sources, and not have to have the drug rep——

Dr. WILKES. I am a tad embarrassed to answer your question because the answer is that doctors don't read the medical literature, and somebody who comes in with a free lunch or gift or an invitation to a sporting event, and tells them that this is a better drug than what they are using is a far more powerful message. It should be the other way around; we should read the New England Journal, we should be able to cite that data, but practicing doctors just aren't there.

Mr. WAXMAN. They are relying a lot on what the drug reps have to say.

Dr. WILKES. Enormously. I think that 90 percent——

Mr. WAXMAN. Let me ask Dr. Erb about that. Why would Merck instruct its sales force not to discuss the results of the VIGOR study with doctors?

Mr. ERB. Well, let me first state we widely disclosed the results of the VIGOR study, as you just indicated: through the press release, through a scientific forum, and also through the New England Journal of Medicine. We believe that it did get wide and broad pickup——

Mr. WAXMAN. Well, maybe it did, but if a doctor heard something about an article in the New England Journal of Medicine, you are the drug rep from Merck, I heard about this, what do you know about it, and that representative is instructed not to answer the question, say I can't even talk about it.

Mr. ERB. The representative is instructed to, if it is an unsolicited question from the physician, that they can send in what we call a professional information request, and information will be sent to the physician based on that question. This is in concert with our commitment that we promote our products based on the currently approved label; and VIGOR, at that point in time, wasn't approved. But physicians did have a method of getting that information, and as I mentioned before——

Mr. WAXMAN. So, in other words——

Mr. ERB [continuing]. With 123,000 PIR requests, we feel that it was fairly widely distributed and people knew about it.

Mr. WAXMAN. So you had it widely distributed, but your representatives were not allowed to mention it because they could take the time, if they want to, to contact your centralized people who will give them an answer. Is that what doctors were supposed to do?

Mr. ERB. In compliance with our commitment to promote information that is in accordance with the approved label and the laws and regulations on those——

Mr. WAXMAN. Well, let us get to the labels.

Mr. ERB [continuing]. We specifically instructed our representatives that they were not allowed to provide information on VIGOR because VIGOR was not part of the approved label at that point in time.

Mr. WAXMAN. OK. Let me take this in two parts. A doctor can go and then contact Merck's centralized authority to get a specific answer. Now, we looked at these documents, and my staff put together from the documents doctors who did contact Merck's medical services department, but didn't get the information they needed. In one letter that was provided to us by a Philadelphia surgeon, Merck presented the data from the cardiovascular card in an even more misleading fashion than the card itself.

If you turn to Document 5, page 4, when this doctor goes to the extra effort to write Merck about the health risks, he gets back the same data that was in the cardiovascular card, except that the placebo column, which showed elevated risks for Vioxx, is now deleted. So I am just wondering why that is the case. Do you have any thoughts on that?

Mr. ERB. I am not familiar with that specific case. What occurs is if a physician has a specific unsolicited question, we have our representatives submit a PIR so that we answer those questions.

Mr. WAXMAN. What is a PIR?

Mr. ERB. That is a professional information request. If it is an unsolicited question, they take that question, send it to headquarters, and headquarters responds with an appropriate response.

Mr. WAXMAN. Well, this is the kind of response that we have heard about that they were getting from this PIR.

Now, the other point you made is that you couldn't talk about VIGOR because it wasn't on the label. Is that what you are telling us?

Mr. ERB. At the time that we are talking about, before it was incorporated into the label, we, in accordance to our programs and policies, we were not allowed to speak about it because the point of VIGOR was to actually change the label. Until we had approved FDA labeling on that change, we were not allowed to communicate.

Mr. WAXMAN. Well, it took a long time before FDA got together with you finally to work out the label change. But you knew from the VIGOR study, you meaning Merck, that there was an increased cardiovascular risk. Why couldn't you tell that to people, even though the VIGOR study was not on the label?

Mr. ERB. I thought I answered that question. Let me explain it again. We widely disseminated the results of the VIGOR trial——

Mr. WAXMAN. No, I understand that.

Mr. ERB [continuing]. Through a press release, scientific forums——

Mr. WAXMAN. But why couldn't you give them the information?

Mr. ERB. We did. If they had an unsolicited question about the VIGOR trial, our professional representatives would fill out a PIR and information would then be sent on the VIGOR trial to those physicians.

Mr. WAXMAN. Now, I want everyone to be clear about the CV card itself, this cardiovascular card. The studies were the same studies from the label, but the analysis of the studies were not on the label, the mortality comparisons were not on the label. How were you able to talk about things that weren't on the label using that CV card, if you are restricted to what is on the label?

Mr. ERB. We promote in accordance to the label. The label is developed by taking all the studies that were part of the original new drug application and summarizing it in a fashion that physicians can use. The information that is in that CV card come from those studies and are consistent with the information that is in the label. Those specific tables, as you have indicated, are not represented on the label, but the data that is on this card are from the exact same studies that were approved.

Mr. WAXMAN. Well, it is not on the label itself. But whether or not VIGOR is on the label I think is irrelevant as a matter of law. We have reviewed the FDA regulations. They don't prevent a pharmaceutical representative from discussing studies that show a drug has a safety risk. They do prevent a drug company from talking about unapproved uses. They do restrict the drug company from saying that a drug is safer than is supported by valid evidence, but they don't prevent a drug company from alerting doctors about new potential safety risks.

That would be an absurd result. It seems to me it is an absurd result for Merck's representatives not to give this information to doctors because they are using the label as a basis for not making the statement.

My time has expired, but I will have other questions when we come back.

Chairman TOM DAVIS. Thank you very much.

Mr. Gutknecht.

Mr. GUTKNECHT. Thank you, Mr. Chairman.

I am having trouble kind of finding my way through all of this. Apparently, if it not on the label, you can't discuss it; and if it is on the label—this is just confusing and, in fact, in some respects, embarrassing.

I want to call the committee's attention to something that the FDA is putting out in large quantities today. It is a little card, and on the front it says "Looking can be deceiving. The medicine you buy from outside the United States may be unsafe or ineffective. Don't risk your health." I want to submit this for the record because the FDA is spending an awful lot of time and trouble and money——

Chairman TOM DAVIS. Without objection, it will go in the record.

Mr. GUTKNECHT [continuing]. Warning people about buying their drugs from Canada, where they can save anywhere from 50 to 200 percent.

On the other hand, the FDA seems to be uninterested in the fact that—and part of the reason we are here today, Dr. Graham, who did the biggest study on Vioxx, testified before the Senate Finance Committee that he believed that Vioxx contributed to as many as 139,000 heart attacks and killed as many as 55,000 people.

Now, we have asked the FDA several times how many people have died from taking drugs that they bought in Canada. The answer is easy to remember, it is a nice round number: it is zero. And yet the FDA is putting out literature like this and they are playing see no evil, speak no evil on the issue of these Cox–2 inhibitors.

Dr. Erb, I want to come back to something you volunteered in the first part of your testimony. You said that your father had taken one of these Cox–2 inhibitors and had stopped taking it. Why did he stop taking it?

Mr. ERB. Vioxx was withdrawn from the marketplace. We voluntarily withdrew it in September.

Mr. GUTKNECHT. Now that there are other Cox–2 inhibitors back on the market is he going to start taking them again?

Mr. ERB. My father's discussion of what he is going to take I think is between he and his physician.

Mr. GUTKNECHT. That is a very good point, it is between he and his physician. But don't you assume that the physician is getting accurate information about the drugs that he may be prescribing for your father or my father or someone else's father?

Mr. ERB. To my knowledge of how Merck approaches it, I think we are providing accurate and balanced information regarding our products, yes.

Mr. GUTKNECHT. So you believe that the cards that were distributed to your pharmaceutical reps were accurate and fair and provided balanced information to the physicians who were prescribing the drug?

Mr. ERB. Yes, the cards that we are providing are accurate, balanced, and fair.

Mr. GUTKNECHT. Did you personally approve Operation Offense?

Mr. ERB. No, I did not approve Operation—I am not part of that.

Mr. GUTKNECHT. Do you know who did?

Mr. ERB. Not to my knowledge, but we could get that information for you.

Mr. GUTKNECHT. Because it is interesting, too, with all of these memos it always says To:, but it never says from whom, and no one seems to want to take responsibility for putting out information that at least an outside observer might call a little disingenuous.

Do you believe that Operation Offense was really designed to inform physicians and their patients, or was it really designed to help sell more product?

Mr. ERB. We believe that providing balanced——

Mr. GUTKNECHT. No, I didn't ask what we believed, I asked what you believed.

Mr. ERB. I believe that providing accurate and balanced information as we do, and the policies and procedures we have in place to ensure that is very important for physicians. We believe in the value and I believe in the value of our products, and we believe that if physicians understand——

Mr. GUTKNECHT. Listen, I believe in the value of most of your products as well, and I am not here just to beat up on the pharmaceutical industry, but I have to tell you that when I look at these memos and these documents, the principle purpose is not to inform physicians. In fact, at every turn it actually instructs them to bring back this card, which really isn't at the heart of what the matter was all about. I mean, it is a diversion, it is not about telling them the facts about the studies and the potential dangers. At no point do you ever refer to Dr. Graham's study.

So you believe that this was principally designed to inform physicians about potential dangers?

Mr. ERB. Our methods of communicating with physicians have always been to be accurate and balanced on both the risk and the benefits of our products, and we believe that if we inform physicians about the risk and benefits, that they can make an informed decision about whether their product, in this case Vioxx, is appropriate for their patients.

Mr. GUTKNECHT. Unfortunately, my time has almost expired, but I do want to make certain that this gets in the record.

Chairman TOM DAVIS. Without objection.

[The information referred to follows:]

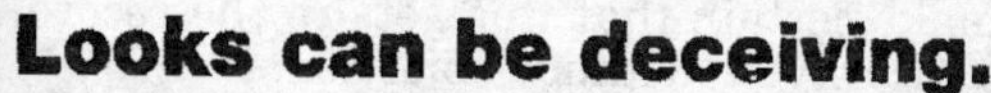

Looks can be deceiving.

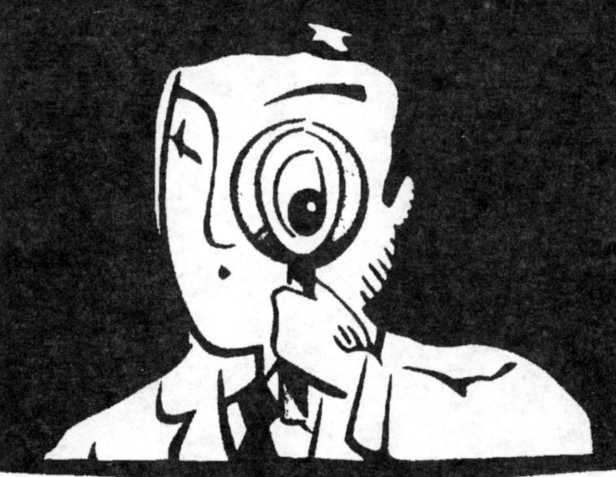

The medicine you buy from
outside the United States
may be unsafe or ineffective.

Don't risk your health.

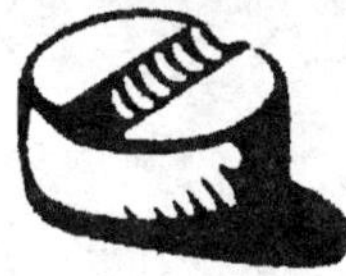

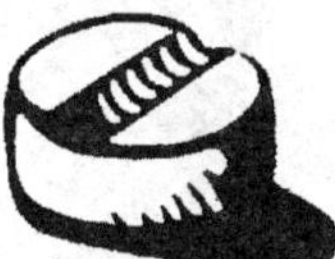

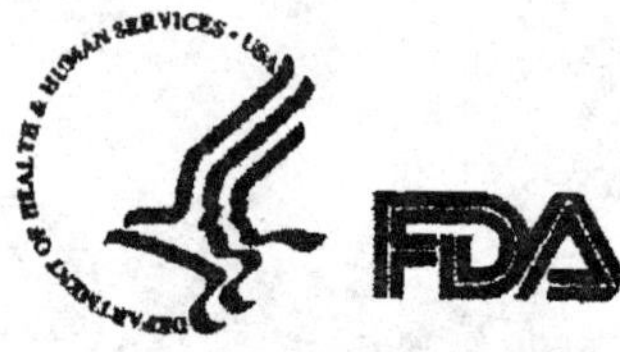

FDA
U.S. Department of Health and Human Services
Food and Drug Administration
www.fda.gov/importeddrugs
1-888-INFO-FDA

Things you should know about buying medicines from outside the United States

If you buy foreign medicine from an Internet site, from a store-front business that offers to order medicine for you, or during visits outside the United States, you are taking a risk. The U.S. Food and Drug Administration (FDA) cannot guarantee the safety of these medicines.

- **QUALITY ASSURANCE CONCERNS.** Medicines that have not been approved for sale in the United States may not have been manufactured under quality assurance procedures designed to produce a safe and effective product.

- **COUNTERFEIT POTENTIAL.** Some imported medicines— even those that bear the name of a U.S.-approved product— may, in fact, be fake versions that are unsafe or even completely ineffective.

- **PRESENCE OF UNTESTED SUBSTANCES.** Some imported medicines and their ingredients, although legal in foreign countries, may not have been evaluated for safety and effectiveness in the United States. These products may be addictive or contain other dangerous ingredients.

- **RISKS OF UNSUPERVISED USE.** Some medicines, whether imported or not, are unsafe when taken without proper medical supervision. You may need a medical evaluation to ensure that the medicine is appropriate for you and your condition. Or, you may require medical checkups to make sure that you are taking the medicine properly, it is working for you, and that you are not having unexpected or life-threatening side effects.

- **LABELING AND LANGUAGE ISSUES.** The medicine's label, including instructions for use and possible side effects, may be in a language you do not understand and may make medical claims or suggest specific uses that have not been properly evaluated for safety and effectiveness.

- **LACK OF INFORMATION.** An imported medicine may lack information that you would need to be promptly and correctly treated for dangerous side effects caused by the medicine.

Remember, medicines you buy from outside the U.S. may be unsafe or ineffective.

It's not worth risking your health!

If you have any questions about the use of any medicines, FDA encourages you to contact your physician, your local pharmacist, or the board of pharmacy for the state in which you live.

(FDA) 04-1511A

Mr. GUTKNECHT. And I would actually hope that at some point we could revisit some of these issues, because while Merck doesn't work for us, and the other pharmaceutical companies don't work for us, the FDA does. And it seems to me that they are shirking their responsibilities to physicians and to consumers in the United States, and many Americans have been harmed because of it. Thank you.

Chairman TOM DAVIS. The pharmaceuticals operate under the rules that we write and the FDA writes, so I think that is appropriate to address it to the FDA.

Mr. GUTKNECHT. But it is clear that the rules are very clumsy, and if the only thing they can inform patients and physicians about are issues that are directly related to the label, then perhaps we ought to take control of those labels away from the pharmaceutical industry and give them to the FDA.

Chairman TOM DAVIS. Thank you.

Mr. Towns.

Mr. TOWNS. Thank you very much, Mr. Chairman.

Dr. Erb, you have been here throughout the morning, right?

Mr. ERB. I was here for the FDA discussions, yes.

Mr. TOWNS. Right. Are the negative marketing practices which have been discussed earlier an accurate reflection of Merck's product marketing strategy?

Mr. ERB. We believe that it is important to promote our products on an accurate and balanced manner. We feel if we do that, and do it in accordance to the approved label, that physicians will understand the value of our drugs and make the appropriate decisions for their patients.

Mr. TOWNS. As part of the post-market surveillance regulations, would you object to greater authority for the Office of New Drugs to require label changes or additional research? Would you object to that?

Mr. ERB. I am not sure I understood your question.

Mr. TOWNS. As part of the post-market surveillance regulations, would you object to greater authority for the Office of New Drugs to require label changes or additional research if they made that request?

Mr. ERB. The FDA right now actually has that ability. They can ask us to do additional studies and can also ask us, if they feel there is a safety issue, to update our label. When we receive a request like that from the FDA, we take it very seriously and we work with them to satisfy those type of requests.

In the situation we are speaking about here on Vioxx, we actually initiated the studies on our own to get a better understanding of the safety profile of the product; we didn't need to be told by the agency to do that. And part of that is through the incentive that we can look at other indications for the drug, and I think it is very important that we have that ability to do it. If the agency felt that there was a safety issue, they could have instructed us to change the label, and we would have taken that very seriously.

Mr. TOWNS. So, in answer, you would not object.

Mr. ERB. I believe they have that ability to do it right now.

Mr TOWNS. But that is not the question. Would you object? You would not object.

Mr. ERB. I don't understand the specific proposal that you are proposing.

Mr. TOWNS. I said would you object to the greater authority for the Office of New Drugs to require—if they have that authority, then you wouldn't object to it, if they have it already.

Mr. ERB. I believe they have that authority right now, to request changes, and they can request changes. In my experience, they have requested changes on products in a class manner; they just did that in April of this year on these Cox–2 inhibitors. They have asked Pfizer to pull one of their products off the marketplace, and they are asking warnings to go on to the NSAIDs. So the agency has that ability to do it today.

Mr. TOWNS. And you don't object. OK.

Do any regulatory agencies in other countries have the authority to mandate label changes or additional research during the post-marketing period? Would you know?

Mr. ERB. In my experience, the other agencies that I have experience with can ask for label changes similar to how FDA asks for it.

Mr. TOWNS. Would you know, Mr. Calfee?

Mr. CALFEE. About other nations?

Mr. TOWNS. Yes.

Mr. CALFEE. I know very little about their regimes. I know that most of them pretty much follow the lead of the FDA, but they occasionally do depart from FDA practices.

Mr. TOWNS. How about you, Dr. Wilkes?

Dr. WILKES. I am only familiar with the UK, and I know that while they collaborate with the FDA, they are quite aggressive about marketing practices. I don't know about in terms of labels, but they are much quicker to act than our FDA is.

Mr. TOWNS. Much quicker.

Dr. WILKES. In the UK.

Mr. TOWNS. Given the new requirements for labeling after an advisory council vote, do you feel comfortable returning Vioxx to the market, particularly given the continuing consumer demand for the product, Dr. Erb?

Mr. ERB. I am sorry, could you repeat the question again?

Mr. TOWNS. Given the new requirements for labeling after the advisory council vote, do you feel comfortable returning Vioxx to the market, particularly given the continuing demand for the product?

Mr. ERB. I believe in the safety of Vioxx. As I mentioned before, we have initiated discussions with the agency with regards to what information they would need to see before allowing Vioxx to go back on the marketplace, but we have not made a decision whether we would do that at this time.

Mr. TOWNS. So I am not sure of your answer. What are you saying, that you feel comfortable?

Mr. ERB. I thought I answered the question. I feel very positive about the safety profile of Vioxx and the unique benefits Vioxx brings, but we are in preliminary discussions with FDA on what information they would like to see with regard to Vioxx before allowing it back on the marketplace. But we have not made a decision at Merck, at this point in time, whether Vioxx would come back onto the marketplace.

Mr. TOWNS. Thank you.

Chairman TOM DAVIS. Thank you very much.

Mr. Souder.

Mr. SOUDER. I thank the chairman.

I want to make a couple comments, then I have a couple questions for Dr. Erb.

First, I think Mr. Calfee raised the dilemma that we face when are trying to move drugs to market, we are trying to help people address different things, whether it is, as we have dealt with, drug abuse in Oxycontin; what does it do to help pain relief; what will happen if people don't have Oxycontin; how do you balance that with those who abuse it.

In this case, of Cox–2 inhibitors, they may save lives in another way, and the question is how do we balance off how many lives are lost, what is full disclosure, and how we go through that process. And I think you added that to the debate of the difficulty of this.

I understand Dr. Wilkes' points, but I do believe it is important for the record that I believe that while you make a good point, you over-exaggerate and demean most doctors in America. Most doctors do not get their advice solely from going out to dinner. And the implication, which I have concerns about as well—and my question is going to get into the marketing question—but most doctors that I know have a multiplicity of ways that they determine this, and it demeans them to imply that their primary way, or that they are going to be inordinately influenced. It is one influencer, and we need to watch that influence, but to demean the doctors as a profession by saying the pharmaceutical reps are determining what they prescribe, when it is one part of what they prescribe, I think is unfair to doctors as a whole.

Into the specific questions with Dr. Erb, I have a technical question and then goes beyond this. One of the key things here seems to be that in your first study, basically, you appear to have concluded that the adverse events were basically different in Vioxx because some of the people were using naproxen to disguise, basically it would be like an aspirin type thing that was fighting off the heart disease, and you felt that was the reason for the difference. In your statement you said because the placebos didn't show that, you presumed that it was the naproxen that was giving the different results.

However, in the letter of warning that came from the Department of Health and Human Services, they specifically said that there are no adequate or well controlled studies of naproxen to support your assertion that naproxen's transient inhibition was true. They also, in this letter, which is not very mild, I mean, in one section they say you minimized, you minimized, you omitted, you promoted for unapproved uses, you promoted unapproved dosing. They are particularly talking about an audio conference. They go through unsubstantiated claims, omission of important risk information.

This was all in 2001, concluding with your minimizing these potential risks and misrepresenting the safety profile of Vioxx raised significant public health and safety questions. And argue we have argued about this card, that it falsely compared; you exaggerated, you downplayed, you didn't have evidence. And given the fact that some of us feel they weren't aggressive, this is a pretty aggressive letter, even if they didn't do anything.

Here is what my question is. Did you try to isolate naproxen at all before you made that assertion, or did you merely make the assertion because of the placebo? And did you do any followup to see, and is that what your followup study tried to do, was isolate opposite naproxen? And if you in fact knew you were going to do a followup study, why did you make the assertion before you knew it was true?

And this comes to the big question I would like you to address, and that is really what we are fundamentally trying to do here is we try to move more drugs to market faster, which gives us lower cost, gives people all sorts of cures for other types of things, in addition to the risks of those drugs. The real question that the American people want to know, as we are getting into these questions about your agents, whether you are manipulating evidence in these cards, whether you are responding to the letters, is can we trust you?

Ultimately, what internal guards do you have at Merck that say this isn't just about money, it isn't just about whether we are going to be sued; we are not just trying to beat out Celebrex or another company? Because if we, as Members of Congress, say, look, we want to move this stuff faster and we want to have this interaction, we have to know not that it takes 3 more years, but that you are reacting fast, that you have a balance, that it isn't just about profits.

And those of us who support this need to have consumers somewhat relief; otherwise, we have to have the FDA take more aggressiveness. And I didn't feel that they were particularly comforting about what they were doing in the first panel on very difficult questions like this.

Chairman TOM DAVIS. Thank you. The gentleman's time has expired.

Mr. SOUDER. Could I hear a response?

Chairman TOM DAVIS. Sure.

Mr. ERB. Can I respond to that, please?

Congressman, Merck is a data-driven company. We follow the procedures of scientific investigation, openeness and disclosure, and scientific integrity. All the decisions we make—marketing, regulatory and otherwise—are based on scientific data and based on the information that these studies provide. We conducted well controlled clinical trials in order to understand the safety and the benefits of our products. We did so in the Vioxx case. These three principles of scientific investigation, openness and integrity I believe were there every step of the way.

Chairman TOM DAVIS. Thank you very much.

The gentleman from Maryland.

Mr. CUMMINGS. Dr. Wilkes, you heard the testimony. Is this unusual, what Merck has done with regard to this whole—I understand that Merck is not as bad as some other companies.

Dr. WILKES. Right. I have spent 15 years researching in this area, both advertising and promotion to doctors and direct to consumer advertising, and to answer your second question, I do think that Merck has a higher standard and is better respected by physicians than most of pharmaceutical companies. To answer your first question, it is not at all unusual that this type of inaccurate information would be palmed off on physicians under the guise of education.

Mr. CUMMINGS. Mr. Chairman, those who manufacture Bextra and Celebrex, are we going to call them in too, in fairness to Merck? Are we going to have another hearing on this? Because I do want to be fair to Merck, because I am getting ready to ask them some questions in a minute.

Chairman TOM DAVIS. Well, let me just say I think it is very clear that what Merck has done is not out of line with industry. Now, Mr. Waxman and I will discuss that.

Mr. CUMMINGS. Well, I hope so, on behalf of my——

Mr. WAXMAN. Would the gentleman yield to me?

Mr. CUMMINGS. Yes, I certainly will.

Mr. WAXMAN. I think it is important that we not just have Merck, but we hear from these other companies as well. We ought to get the documents from them and then talk about another hearing, because we have to, I think, give a more balanced picture than just have one company.

Chairman TOM DAVIS. Merck, by and large, has been a very good company.

Mr. CUMMINGS. Yes, that is fine. But I want to know about— Merck, you don't produce Celebrex, do you? No? I will answer it for you. You don't produce Bextra, do you?

Mr. ERB. No, we don't.

Mr. CUMMINGS. You don't produce Bextra. I want to know about them. We just heard Dr. Wilkes say that the other companies are worse, so we really need to hear from them. And I am looking forward to that, Mr. Chairman. My constituents are anxiously waiting to hear that testimony, and I am too.

Let me just go to you, Dr. Erb. Let me ask you this. You know, I have been reading some of this material, and you apparently have a video, and it blows my mind. It says, "Let's listen to part of Martin Luther King's I have a dream speech." Then you show the video. Then it says, "King was someone who was goal focused. He kept getting shut down, but he kept going. How many times did he repeat the phrase 'I have a dream'?" And then they go on to say, "Just as with the physician, you must keep repeating the compelling message. At some point the physician will be free at last when he or she prescribes the Merck drug that is the most appropriate for the patient."

Is that the way you all sell these drugs? Is that what you teach these salespersons to do?

Mr. ERB. What we teach our salespersons to do is to follow the policies and procedures that we have in place.

Mr. CUMMINGS. Is this a part of the policies and procedures?

Mr. ERB. I am confident that those policies and procedures, and our training methods for them, ensure that our representatives present to physicians the information in a fair and balanced manner, and that it is accurate. I am not familiar with the documents that you are reading from.

Mr. CUMMINGS. Let me tell you another one, because you might want to get familiar. Part of your procedure—this is a part of the training—says "Helen Keller could have felt sorry for herself when she went blind and deaf. Martin Luther King could have laid low when his home was firebombed. Tiger Woods could have avoided the pressure by not turning pro as young as he did." And then you went all the way back to George Washington: "George Washington could have finished his years with a comfortable life without the challenges of taking on the Presidency."

Just so that you will have that. I know you want to look it up, because that is a part of what the Merck's training program is all about. And I just want to make sure that when these doctors are being convinced of things and to prescribe these drugs, that they are about the business of prescribing the things that are best for our constituents.

I am tired of people dying because of prescriptions that they should have never been prescribed, and in some kind of way we have to get control over that. And then when I see things like this, Martin Luther King, my God. How far will we go?

So I will yield the rest of my time to Mr. Waxman, Mr. Chairman.

Mr. WAXMAN. Well, thank you. Just 20 seconds.

On the question of what we do with the other companies, Mr. Chairman, I think we ought to get the documents from these other companies. Whether we hold a hearing or not, that is something we ought to discuss later. But I think it would be helpful for this committee to get the documents, especially for those companies that we don't even think of in the same high caliber that we think of Merck itself.

Chairman TOM DAVIS. I think we can do that. We obviously have other priorities right now, but we can get the documents and look at them and work our way through.

Mr. WAXMAN. Thank you very much.

Chairman TOM DAVIS. Thank you.

Mr. Lynch.

Mr. LYNCH. Thank you, Mr. Chairman. I want to thank you and the ranking member for your work on this issue.

Dr. Erb, if I could ask you. I have this very strong concern about going beyond the individual physician with the direct advertising to the public, and I am looking at Document No. 17 which you have provided to the committee. I guess the page number is 586. The document explains that Merck not only pinpoints a doctor's current prescribing, but also assigns a Merck potential that is a dollar amount of Merck drugs that she or he should be prescribing, and bonuses are tied to realizing the "Merck potential number."

Given the fact that the advertising that you are doing is going past the physician, directly to the consumer, to ask for a certain drugs, and then putting the additional pressure on that physician to meet a certain number, is that good? Is that good for the general public? Is it circumventing the responsibility that we thought we gave to the doctors to make these decisions? And if we spent—I think the number is $300 million—$300 million—and I understand Mr. Calfee's suggestion that even though you spent $300 million to convince people what to buy, that it had no effect. I certainly think I have a different view of things.

But can you tell me, isn't this circumventing the physician's role? Isn't this treating these pharmaceuticals as just one other commodity, where the program is just sell, sell, sell, with the real benefit to the consumer becoming secondary? I would like to hear your response.

Mr. ERB. We believe that direct to consumer advertising actually has a benefit in that it increases the public's awareness of disease states, therapeutic options that they may have. We believe that this will result in more patients seeking appropriate diagnosis and treatment of their medicines. It is to that avenue that we feel that it is important to have direct to consumer advertising.

Mr. LYNCH. And you don't think you are overstepping that physician's role to prescribe by going directly to the consumer and marketing this thing in such a commercial way?

Mr. ERB. No, we don't think we are overstepping the physician's role, because the patient would have to then contact their physician and seek their medical input.

Mr. LYNCH. Dr. Wilkes, what do you think about this?

Dr. WILKES. I think it is naive. I think that there is an enormous amount of pressure that is placed on the physician. More and more we are being evaluated by patient satisfaction surveys. It is extremely difficult to say no to a patient who comes in and asks you for a drug. If it is totally inappropriate, none of us would prescribe a totally dangerous drug, but we often prescribe drugs that we are in the middle of the road about because of the pressure from the patient.

And I have just published a study in the Journal of the American Medical Association last week that looked at this and showed that when patients come in and ask for a specific drug, they are more often likely to get that drug than when they come in and talk about the symptoms they are less likely to get a drug.

Mr. LYNCH. Right. It appears to be almost self-prescribing when they are walking in and saying, I want this drug.

Now, the argument that this $300 million that is being spent to directly convince the consumer to ask for a specific drug, it has been suggested here this morning that had no effect.

Dr. WILKES. I think the data shows otherwise. And perhaps your allusion or reference to the fact that no industry in this country is going to spend that kind of money without absolute clear data that it is working just because we don't have the data, that data is proprietary and isn't shared with us. But they are not going to be that foolish to keep, year after year—and the money increases, it doesn't decrease.

Mr. LYNCH. Right. Well, thank you.

Thank you, Mr. Chairman.

Chairman TOM DAVIS. Thank you very much.

I think we are going to do just 5 more minutes on each side.

Mr. Calfee, Dr. Wilkes states in his testimony that pharmaceutical promotion and direct to consumer advertising has an impact on doctors' prescribing behavior. In the case of Vioxx, what effect did promotional materials and DTC advertising have on physician's prescribing?

Mr. CALFEE. We know little about that, we don't know a lot. I think the fact that the companies actually spend a very small amount on DTC advertising in comparison to total sales strongly suggests that the advertising itself was not generating very large returns. I think there are persuasive reasons to think that DTC advertising was a relatively small factor in the growth of this particular market. The Cox–2s did well in other countries where there was no DTC advertising whatsoever.

I think we have to remember that what a DTC ad does is it said to a patient, it said essentially if you are in pain, there is a drug you can take that may relieve your pain. If you are already taking a drug, there is another one that may relieve it better, and you can talk to your doctor about that.

Chairman TOM DAVIS. The pharmaceutical reps, Dr. Erb, they are not technical people, they are not doctors for the most part, is that right? I mean, they are out there to make sales. Giving the a larger burden to try to explain things back and forth, does that incur some difficulty, when you get them too technical?

Mr. ERB. We train our sales force to speak about our medicines and use approved materials that are consistent with the label, so we do extensive training with the sales force to make sure that they are representing the information about our products in an accurate and balanced manner.

Chairman TOM DAVIS. On the Vioxx side, you had how many physicians would call up or go to your Web site to get additional information besides what the sales rep were hearing? You gave a number prior to this, I think.

Mr. ERB. Yes. I was referring to the professional information requests. These are unsolicited requests that physicians make to our sales force. And what we do is then provide to our headquarters that question, and they respond with appropriate information regarding the request from the physician.

Chairman TOM DAVIS. How detailed would they get with that physician?

Mr. ERB. They will answer the question consistently as to what the physician is looking for. It can get into some significant detail that is appropriate for what the physician was asking.

Chairman TOM DAVIS. And obviously thousands of physicians avail themselves of that because they had concerns based on published reports and wanted to understand it.

Mr. ERB. Correct. I think regarding the VIGOR findings, they were widely distributed, and I think you can see that 123,000 requests is quite a large number, so they were very well informed of what was going on.

Chairman TOM DAVIS. And a sales rep, even though you educate them, they give them talking points, some of the intricacies that they would be asked on this would probably go beyond their level of understanding, wouldn't it?

Mr. ERB. It possibly would. They are trained to make sure that they stay within the information that is approved in the prescribing information, so they have to use materials that have been approved, that go through our medical legal group, which is two physicians and a lawyer, to ensure that the material is appropriate and balanced and consistent with the label, and they are to stay within that material and consistent with the label.

Chairman TOM DAVIS. Thank you.

Dr. Wilkes, you mentioned in your testimony that education of physicians on how to appropriately prescribe pharmaceuticals really should begin in medical school, that this is a shortcoming of society and, as a result of that, companies are able to use the rules that are written in a manner which you prefer that they didn't. As vice dean for medical education at UC-Davis, what specific actions have you taken there to improve physician education prior to graduation and residency?

Dr. WILKES. Well, two major steps. One is that we prohibit our students from having any contact at all with pharmaceutical reps, period, zero, none.

The second is that we do have an exercise in the third year of medical school whereby we have our clinical pharmacists come in as drug reps and give a demonstration to the students and talk with them. The students do a survey before and after this sham procedure, and then we dissect apart what they told us, what the evidence was, how they pitched it to the doctors so that the doctors are better consumers of this information.

We are using pharmacists, many of whom had previously been detailers; not for Merck, but for all of the different companies. So they are all pharmacists at the hospital now, but they have a prior life as drug detailers.

Chairman TOM DAVIS. And although you would like to have pharmaceutical advertising presentations be different than they are, in point of fact, a well informed doctor who is subject to that can make a huge difference for the patient, can't they?

Dr. WILKES. They do. And perhaps I can take a second and address the Congressman's concern before. When I said that doctors overwhelmingly learn about drugs from the pharmaceutical companies, he took it to mean from detailers. The committee should understand that the manufacturers have a huge influence over what gets published in journals.

The journals are filled with drug ads; lectures are sponsored by pharmaceutical companies; detailers visit doctors; doctors requesting formulary additions to the hospitals; and, last, the manufacturers are giving free samples to doctors, which patients love. So all of these things combined are an enormous—I mean, probably 95 percent of the influence on doctors' prescribing comes from the pharmaceutical company, not from any independent source.

Chairman TOM DAVIS. But I will just take a second, if the committee will indulge me.

In this case, as soon as they had been through their VIGOR test, they released this to the public, there were medical results published, and that became an important part of the decisionmaking.

Dr. WILKES. Right. Again——

Chairman TOM DAVIS. As opposed to attempting to hide it or something.

Dr. WILKES. Absolutely. The problem is not so much that I have seen any attempt to hide this or keep it from the doctors. The problem is that we don't have an effective dissemination arm. NIH issues guidelines, the cholesterol education program issues guidelines. Doctors don't follow guidelines; they don't keep up. And it is not necessarily, in that sense, the pharmaceutical companies' fault, but we need a better way to have doctors practicing based on evidence that is scientifically sound.

Chairman TOM DAVIS. Point well taken. Thank you.

Mr. Waxman.

Mr. WAXMAN. Just to follow on that point, Dr. Wilkes, Dr. Erb said that what they are trying to do is give a fair and balanced presentation from the sales representative to the doctor. Yet, that presentation is not going to be talking about the results of the VIGOR study, after the VIGOR study had been done and after it had been published. Is it fair and balanced not to talk about the VIGOR study?

Dr. WILKES. With all due respect, I disagree very strongly with Mr. Erb. I think that the VIGOR study is a vital study. It was the biggest study applied most directly to patients that take Vioxx. Most patients don't take Vioxx, as someone said, for a few days for an ankle injury, they take it for months and months and months; and those are the patients who take higher doses, and those are the patients that we need to worry about. And that VIGOR study should have been an essential part of what they were talking about.

Mr. WAXMAN. Well, the other part of Dr. Erb's position is that it has to be fair and balanced, but consistent with the label. Now, in your booklet, Document 9, in this document Merck told their representatives you can't talk about what the FDA said about the VIGOR study, but Merck allowed its representatives to say that VIGOR "was an 8,000 patient study designed to evaluate the GI safety of Vioxx compared to naproxen. All of the primary endpoints were met."

What do you think Merck is communicating when it says all the primary endpoints were met in the VIGOR study?

Dr. WILKES. I think they are probably trying to have it both ways. I am not sure, perhaps Dr. Erb can address what they actually meant, but it seems to me that they are contradicting themselves.

Mr. WAXMAN. Well, Dr. Erb, are you contradicting yourself? You can't talk about the VIGOR study on the cardiovascular, but then you allow your representatives to talk about the VIGOR study meeting all the primary endpoints.

Mr. ERB. Congressman Waxman, what page are you reading from?

Mr. WAXMAN. That is on 1179, Tab 9. Tab 9, page 1179. This is a script. I just read in the news, the doctor says to the representative—I will read it aloud. "I just read in the news that there is a concern about Vioxx and the incidents of heart attacks." And then you are supposed to say, "Doctor, what you may be referring to is a press report addressing the Vioxx GI Outcomes trial, VIGOR, reviewed at the FDA's Arthritis Advisory Committee meeting. This was an 8,000 patient study designed to evaluate the GI safety of Vioxx compared to the NSAID naproxen. All of the primary endpoints were met. However, because the study is not on the label, I cannot discuss the study with you. I would be happy to submit your questions to the medical services department."

Mr. ERB. Right. And the medical services department request is what I was describing before as the professional information request. So if the physician did have a question about VIGOR, we would handle it in that way. But the sales representative, because the labeling had not been approved yet for VIGOR, they were not able to speak about the study.

Mr. WAXMAN. Well, the labeling hadn't been approved for VIGOR at all; yet, you are allowing the sales reps to talk about VIGOR where it makes a positive statement about the drug.

And I gather what they mean by primary endpoints is the GI issues, is that right, Dr. Wilkes?

Dr. WILKES. That is how I would interpret it. Remember, none of these drugs, none of the Cox–2 drugs, have ever been shown to be more effective than aspirin, so the only benefit they have is in the GI arena. So that would be my assumption as well.

Mr. WAXMAN. What do you say about that, Dr. Erb?

Mr. ERB. The primary endpoints were GI outcome endpoints, that is correct.

Mr. WAXMAN. OK. Well, it seems to me, the way I see the problem, Merck has permitted its representatives to provide information outside of its label regarding the benefit of its drugs, but not the risks, and I don't think that is providing education to doctors. It is misleading, it withholds from them the information that they most need to know, which is whether Vioxx is dangerous.

Now, the cardiovascular card that you instructed your reps to show, Merck tried to get that on the label and FDA said no. FDA said we are not going to put that on the label. Even though you tried to get it on the negotiations, FDA said the company sought to put the label data from Vioxx preapproval studies, the same studies summarized in the cardiovascular card that the company representatives have been showing to physicians for 2 years, FDA rejected Merck's proposal. So you tried to get it on and FDA said no.

If I might just one further question, Mr. Chairman. I do want to just touch on an issue, and I know we are running out of time.

Dr. Erb, there is a recent New York Times article that discussed Merck documents that indicated the company developed a plan in 1999 to neutralize influential physicians who were not supporters of Vioxx. According to the article, it appeared from the documents that Merck had offered grants and travel to these physicians to alter their opinions of Vioxx. Can you explain what was going on? What does that mean, neutralizing a physician?

Mr. ERB. What it means is that we feel that when physicians have either lack of information or misinformation about our products, that it is important to make sure that they have full understanding of both the benefits and limitations of our products. And the intent here is to provide them that education so we can bring them back to a more neutral and balanced position about our product when they consider it for their patients.

Mr. WAXMAN. Dr. Wilkes, do you have any feelings about that?

Dr. WILKES. Well, I think that this isn't about neutralizing, it is about swaying and making their suspicions or concerns not concerns, and it is to mislead them and downplay what they are feeling are major concerns about something that might impact on their patients. This isn't neutralizing, it is worse than that.

Mr. WAXMAN. Well, Mr. Chairman, maybe there is nothing wrong with the effort to neutralize physicians, but it seems that something more——

Mr. DENT [presiding]. You don't have any more time.

Mr. WAXMAN. Well, let me complete my sentence. Unfortunately, Mr. Davis isn't here, and my request is really to him. But it seems like it is something learning more about, and I would like to have the chairman, when he comes back, have the committee send a document request on this issue of neutralizing physicians, because I want to know more about it; what it means actually to neutralize doctors. Thank you.

Mr. DENT. Thank you, Mr. Waxman. The chairman will return momentarily.

Thank you, gentlemen, for being here this afternoon. I apologize for not being here sooner. Prior to coming to the Congress, I served as an acting chairman of the consumer protection licensure committee in my State, so I spent a lot of time on patient safety and consumer protection issues. On a more parochial level, I represent a county in Congress where Merck has over 10,000 employees, over 1,500 of whom reside in my congressional district. So I wanted to just put that out there on the record.

I guess the question I have is for Dr. Erb and then for Mr. Calfee. As we look at weighing the risks versus the benefits as to effective pain relief medication versus possible cardiovascular risks, how do we as a Congress, or as an FDA, especially, make that calculation, the risk versus the benefit? Because since Merck pulled that Vioxx off the market, I know there were many patients across the country who wanted that product, they wanted that pain relief; and it was very important to them and they were willing to accept the cardiovascular risk associated with Vioxx. Could you respond to that, Dr. Erb, and then maybe Mr. Calfee?

Mr. ERB. Yes. I think the best way to assess the benefit and risk is to thoroughly look through the data from the files, and the complete set of data and the weight of evidence; and that is what is presented and disclosed to FDA, who then determines whether the drug is safe and effective before it puts it on the marketplace. We also think it is very important that this information be presented in a balanced fashion and communicated in the label, as well as in other forms, so that physicians can take this information into consideration.

But, in the end, the physician has to decide, based on this information, whether the drug is going to be appropriate for their specific patient. We want to get that information out there to them; we want to make sure it is appropriate and balanced. The FDA wants to make sure in their minds that the risks or the side effect profile and the benefits balance such that it is favorable to put the product onto the marketplace, and they make that determination when they approve the drug.

Mr. DENT. Thank you.

Mr. Calfee.

Mr. CALFEE. I would direct your attention to the FDA memo by Jenkins and Seligman that was released on April 7th. It is really an excellent review of all the evidence, and basically where they come down now, as opposed to the news stories that came out on last September 30th and immediately afterwards in some of the medical journals, is that it looks like the Cox–2s are probably no more dangerous than the NSAIDs, but the NSAIDs themselves may or may not carry some cardiovascular risk.

What we really don't know very much about right now is whether or not there is some probably small risk associated with NSAIDs generally. But right now there doesn't seem to be a whole lot of reason to avoid using the Cox–2s. I think, myself, it is unfortunate that the patients don't have the choice of Vioxx right now.

Mr. DENT. In response to the criticism following the withdrawal of Vioxx, the FDA announced the creation of Drug Safety Monitoring Board. Mr. Calfee, how effective do you think the Drug Safety Monitoring Board will be in monitoring drug safety information and resolving drug safety disputes?

Mr. CALFEE. It remains to be seen. The Board may make some difference. The FDA is going to get some input from outside their agency that they didn't get before. My own view is that the FDA was not very far off the mark on the Vioxx episode. I think they recognized very early that the issue was NSAIDs, and not just Vioxx alone, and they have handled it pretty well.

I guess I have a lot less criticism than some people do to make of how the FDA has been handling drug safety. It is far from perfect. The new Board may improve things to some extent, but it is a very, very tough task, and we will just have to see whether they really get better at it.

Mr. DENT. What kind of lasting impact will the Vioxx episode have on the organizational and regulatory structure at the FDA?

Mr. CALFEE. Well, again, we don't know. I think that the unfortunate fallout here is that the Vioxx episode has demonstrated to the FDA once again that if there are safety questions about drugs they approved, they are going to suffer severe penalties in the form of hearings, adverse publicity, criticism, etc. Whereas, if they are a little bit slower, even quite a bit slow to approve innovative drugs that are still in the pipeline, they don't get very much criticism at all.

I think they are innately conservative; they innately give a great deal of emphasis, a great deal of weight to drug safety, probably too much weight, at least sometimes, and I think that this episode is probably going to reinforce that tendency. My fear is that it will have at least a modest, if not significant, impact in the sense of slowing down the approval of innovative new drugs.

Mr. DENT. Thank you, gentleman, for your testimony, and I will turn back the chair to the Chairman. My time has expired.

Chairman TOM DAVIS [presiding]. Mr. Lynch.

Mr. LYNCH. Thank you, Mr. Chairman.

Chairman TOM DAVIS. Let me just note we have a vote going on, and given other business, we will try to get everybody in before we have to go over for a vote. There is 10 minutes left, so I don't know if anybody else has anything.

Mr. LYNCH. I will try to be quick.

Chairman TOM DAVIS. We are going to try to release this panel at that time.

Mr. Lynch. All right. I will try, Mr. Chairman.

Gentlemen, could you please turn to Document 25? And I think that is page 1307, at the bottom. This course is called "Join the Club" and explains Merck's policy on reprints. Just to bring everybody up to speed, reprints are basically Xeroxed copies of articles that appear, for example, in the New England Journal of Medicine or other prominent journal, about the risks and benefits of particular drugs.

Now, Merck, according to its policy, divides these reprinted articles into two categories. One category is approved reprints, which provides solid evidence as to why customers should be prescribed Merck products for appropriate patients; and then the other reprints that are categorized under the Merck policy are "background reprints," which may not—may not—as a matter of company policy, be distributed to doctors.

Now, Mr. Waxman spoke about fair and balanced communications with doctors, and Dr. Erb talked about appropriate and balanced communication with doctors. What this implies is that if there are two similar studies that reach different conclusions, Merck representatives are directed to distribute one, but are forbidden—forbidden by company policy—from distributing the other.

Now, this is an interesting issue because I have heard some people ask what could possibly be wrong with a drug company representative handing out a scientific paper. If companies are so dramatically skewing, however, the research and the information that they are willing to discuss and share with the customer and with the doctors, it seems to me that doctors and customers, patients, will be mislead.

Mr. Erb, I would like you to respond to the practice, and, Mr. Wilkes, I would like to ask you what are the implications of this policy on just a communicative and a medical education standpoint.

Dr. Erb.

Mr. Erb. Yes. The approved reprints are reprints that are for studies that make up the basis of the label, as well as are consistent with the label. The background information we feel it is very important that our sales reps understand what is happening out in the scientific field at that point in time because the physicians are also keeping up with it.

But in compliance with our policies and practices around promotion and that it has to be consistent with the label, in those cases, if it is not consistent with the label, they are used for their own background, their own information, but they are not instructed to provide that to the physicians.

Mr. Lynch. And you still think that if you are presenting the benefits without emphasizing another article that might emphasize the risks or the negative aspects, if a review is negative, you think it is perfectly fair and balanced to withhold the negative report and present the positive one, is that what you are saying?

Mr. Erb. Our policies and procedures are in place that we present accurate and balanced information regarding the product, so we don't go one side or the other with regards to benefit and risks; we make sure that the information is accurate and is balanced and is consistent with the label.

Mr. Lynch. Consistent with the label. OK.

Dr. Wilkes.

Dr. WILKES. I think that one has to ask what balanced means. I mean, is balanced what is best for the corporate stockholders or is balanced best what is for the patient? You had mentioned that they can't give out the abstract. As I read this document, it says that they can't even discuss the document. And remember that many of these detailers are pharmacists, so they are not just salesmen; they have some scientific background, and they read the literature. A doctor says, well, what about this study? Can't talk about it, you will have to wait until it is officially approved. It is hardly balanced information.

Mr. LYNCH. No. And you are absolutely right, I misspoke. They are not only not allowed to distribute it, they are not allowed to discuss it. So it is an embargo, it is basically precluding any discussion of the matter at all, which I think makes the matter more egregious. Thank you, Doctor.

Thank you, Mr. Chairman.

Chairman TOM DAVIS. Thank you.

Mr. Cummings, you have a couple of minutes.

Mr. CUMMINGS. Thank you very much, Mr. Chairman.

One of the things, Dr. Wilkes, that is very interesting, on Document 18, page 1601, they say this slide is used to teach representatives how to use nonverbal techniques involving the eyes, head, fingers, hands, legs, and overall posture, facial expressions and mirroring. My goodness.

I guess I am trying to figure out, does that bother you at all? I mean, it seems to me—and, again, we are talking about life and death, we are not just talking about a little play thing. We are talking about life and death in some instances. It seems to me that if I have a medication that can do all the things that Merck says it can do and whatever, that I should not have to go through all of this, just present the facts.

Like the thing said, just the facts, ma'am. Just the facts. I shouldn't have to be making these facial expressions and going through all these conniptions. How do you see this, Doctor?

Dr. WILKES. Well, as a doctor, I see it as very demeaning. I mean, I didn't mention before, but this concept of neutralizing—I don't know if you were here for it—that is demeaning. I don't want to be neutralized. And the fact that they have all these tools suggests that this is not education, this is social manipulation. I mean, they have studied this and know exactly how to maximize doctors prescribing the way they want it prescribed.

Mr. CUMMINGS. You heard the comments on Martin Luther King, did you not?

Dr. WILKES. I did.

Mr. CUMMINGS. What did you think of that, same thing?

Dr. WILKES. Absolutely. And Helen Keller and George Washington. I mean, it sounded more like a football rally, you know, what the coach would tell you before you go out for the game, than it did about how we are going to improve the public's health, how we are going to make people's pain go away and make sure that they are safe and healthy.

Mr. CUMMINGS. Mr. Chairman, I know we are running out of time. I yield back.

Chairman TOM DAVIS. Thank you very much.

Let me thank this panel very much for being with us. We will hold the record open for 10 days, and the committee stands adjourned.

Mr. WAXMAN. Mr. Chairman, I also want to join you in thanking the panel and you for holding this hearing. I mentioned this business of getting documents on neutralizing physicians. I think our staffs are talking to each other about that, and I hope will continue to explore it. I think it is an important issue.

Chairman TOM DAVIS. Thank you very much.

[Whereupon, at 1:46 p.m., the committee was adjourned.]

[The prepared statements of Hon. Jon C. Porter and Hon. Lynn A. Westmoreland follow:]

CONGRESSMAN JON C. PORTER
GOVERNMENT REFORM COMMITTEE
"Risk and Responsibility: The Roles of FDA and Pharmaceutical Companies in
Ensuring the Safety of Approved Drugs, Like Vioxx"
May 5, 2005

Mr. Chairman, thank you for holding this hearing today. I would also like to thank all of the witnesses for coming here today to better educate us on this important issue.

Mr. Chairman, the subject of this hearing—the roles of the Food and Drug Administration (FDA) and Pharmaceutical Companies in ensuring the safety of approved drugs—affects millions upon millions of Americans every day.

When a prescription is given by a doctor, and later filled by a pharmacist, Americans trust that what they are taking is safe and will work toward the improvement of their health. Most of these same people are aware that the drugs they are taking may have side effects, and they are given specific instructions on how to take the drug so that adverse reactions are avoided.

What most Americans do not think about, however, is how the drug was determined to be "safe" and what tests have been, and will be, done in order to ensure their safety. They simply believe in the integrity of their pharmacists, physicians, the FDA and the drug companies from which their prescription came.

The recent pulling of major pharmaceutical drugs, such as Vioxx and Bextra, off the market has shaken the public's trust in both the FDA and drug companies. Mr. Chairman, as Members of Congress, it is our job to make sure that the pharmaceutical drug system works and that the public's confidence in approved pharmaceutical drugs is restored.

I am curious to learn more about the relationship between the Office of New Drugs and the Office of Drug Safety, as well as the structure of the Center for Drug Evaluation and Research within the FDA. Specifically, I would like to gain a better understanding as to how the FDA approaches the post-marketing surveillance of drugs, and how the FDA's new Drug Safety Monitoring Board plans on improving this process.

Again, Mr. Chairman, thank you for holding this hearing today. I would also like to thank the witnesses for being here to discuss this issue today. Your expertise and experience is much appreciated. I look forward to working with the Government Reform Committee on this issue.

***

Opening Statement of Rep. Lynn Westmoreland
(GA-08)

before the

Committee on Government Reform

Hearing on Risk and Responsibility: The Roles of FDA and Pharmaceutical
Companies in Ensuring the Safety of Approved Drugs, Like Vioxx

May 5, 2005

Thank you, Mr. Chairman, for holding this important hearing on drug safety. Our nation's drug safety system is vitally important and I appreciate the willingness of the witnesses to testify today on such an important issue.

The federal government has an important responsibility to help make sure drugs are safe for consumers.

But we also must never forget the issue of personal responsibility.

Our knowledge of drugs and their benefits to the human body has increased dramatically over this century, but we are continuing to learn.

Sometimes problems arise that we weren't even capable of knowing when the drug was approved, and other times there are things we can know.

Each drug carries its own unique risk, and those who take them should be able to make the choice, along with input from their physician, regarding the decision to take a drug that may have risks associated with it.

We can't design a test that can predict every single thing that can go wrong with a drug. As much as we would like to, we don't have that ability at this point.

We also need to look at how fears of litigation may keep products off the market that are beneficial for everyone.

After Merck voluntarily removed Vioxx from the market, a cottage industry of lawyers advocating Vioxx claims has sprung up, even as the FDA continues its review of the drug class.

A simple web search can bring up hundreds of websites with information on how to get money from lawsuits regarding Vioxx from lawyers across the country.

I am looking forward to hearing from the witnesses on how and when Merck reacted to the information it had and also how the FDA responded to the information it had.

I am also interested in hearing about how the drug safety process works within the FDA after a drug has received approval.

Thanks to all of you for being here, and we look forward to your testimony.

Thank you, Mr. Chairman.